SELF-ASSES
DIAGNOSTIC

# SELF-ASSESSMENT IN
# Diagnostic Radiology

### Richard M. Mendelson
MB, ChB, MRCP, FRCR
*Senior Lecturer in Diagnostic Radiology*
*University of Liverpool*

### Graham H. Whitehouse
MBBS, FRCP, FRCR, DMRD, AKC
*Professor of Diagnostic Radiology*
*University of Liverpool*

BLACKWELL SCIENTIFIC PUBLICATIONS
OXFORD LONDON EDINBURGH
BOSTON PALO ALTO MELBOURNE

© 1986 by
Blackwell Scientific Publications
Editorial offices:
Osney Mead, Oxford, OX2 0EL
8 John Street, London, WC1N 2ES
23 Ainslie Place, Edinburgh, EH3 6AJ
52 Beacon Street, Boston
   Massachusetts 02108, USA
667 Lytton Avenue, Palo Alto
   California 94301, USA
107 Barry Street, Carlton
   Victoria 3053, Australia

All rights reserved. No part of this
publication may be reproduced,
stored in a retrieval system, or
transmitted, in any form or by any
means, electronic, mechanical,
photocopying, recording or otherwise
without the prior permission of the
copyright owner

First published 1986

Set by Action Typesetting, Gloucester
and printed and bound in Great
Britain by Billing & Sons Ltd,
Worcester.

DISTRIBUTORS

USA
   Blackwell Mosby Book Distributors
   11830 Westline Industrial Drive
   St Louis, Missouri 63141

Canada
   The C.V. Mosby Company
   5240 Finch Avenue East,
   Scarborough, Ontario

Australia
   Blackwell Scientific Publications
      (Australia) Pty Ltd
   107 Barry Street
   Carlton, Victoria 3053

British Library
Cataloguing in Publication Data

Mendelson, Richard M.
   Self assessment in diagnostic
   radiology.
   1. Radiology, Medical—Problems,
   exercises, etc.
   I. Title   II. Whitehouse, G.H.
   616.07'57'076      R896

   ISBN 0-632-01463-6

# Contents

Introduction, vii

## Questions

### Gastrointestinal Tract and Adnexa, 3
Q1–5:    Oesophagus
Q6–7:    Oesophagus/stomach
Q8–13:   Stomach
Q14–18:  Small intestine
Q19–22:  Small/large intestine
Q23–28:  Large intestine
Q29–37:  Biliary tract and liver
Q38–41:  Pancreas
Q42–45:  Miscellaneous

### Locomotor System, 12
Q46–59:  Joint disease
Q60–64:  Spine
Q65–71:  Congenital
Q72–80:  Tumours
Q81–84:  Metabolic bone disease
Q85–93:  Miscellaneous
Q94–95:  Soft tissues

### Genitourinary Tract, 22
Q96–115:   Renal disease
Q116–120:  Bladder and ureters
Q121–123:  Obstetrics
Q124–126:  Gynaecology

### Respiratory System, 29
Q127–132:  Intrinsic/diffuse lung disease
Q133–139:  Lung disease from extrinsic causes
Q140–145:  Neoplasms
Q146–151:  Vascular
Q152–154:  Paediatric
Q155–161:  Miscellaneous

Cardiovascular System, 37
Q162–168: Congenital cardiac disease
Q169–176: Miscellaneous cardiac
Q177–181: Aorta and peripheral vessels

Central Nervous System and Skull, 42
Q182–188: Plain skull
Q189–191: Computed tomography
Q192–196: Miscellaneous

Endocrine System and Metabolism, 46
Q197–201: Adrenals
Q202–204: Thyroid and parathyroid
Q205–211: Miscellaneous

Miscellaneous Topics, 50
Q212–220

**Answers and Notes**

Gastrointestinal Tract and Adnexa, 54
Locomotor System, 83
Genitourinary System, 107
Respiratory System, 129
Cardiovascular System, 153
Central Nervous System and Skull, 167
Endocrine System and Metabolism, 177
Miscellaneous Topics, 186

References, 194

# Introduction

Multiple choice questions nowadays form a large component of the Final Fellowship examination of the Royal College of Radiologists, as well as postgraduate radiological examinations in other parts of the English speaking world. Candidates for the Final Fellowship would inevitably have been exposed to MCQs at earlier stages in their training. Despite this experience, the anticipation of an MCQ paper, with its probing of the recesses of memory and the uncertainties of partial recall, will still strike fear in many seasoned candidates. Inevitably, collections of MCQs have been produced in book form to provide practice in this examination format. When there are merely stark 'yes' or 'no' answers to these questions, the student will find the exercise to be frustrating and of limited value. Explanatory notes to the answers are obviously required in order to give a genuine educative function.

The aims of this particular book are threefold: to test the knowledge of candidates for the Final Fellowship examination and equivalent examinations; to inform; and to provide a guide to further reading. Knowledge is tested by 220 MCQs, set in the same form as that used in the Final Fellowship examination. We have attempted to base the questions on what we generally consider to be important topics in day to day radiological practice, or common subjects in examinations. Obviously not all questions fall into these categories — but any MCQ examination will be a heterogenous mix of common and esoteric topics. In view of the enormous amount of available radiological literature, we have attempted to confine ourselves to key references and review articles. There is a danger that the indolent or pressurized candidate will come to rely on compact books containing concise notes and gamuts. This is obviously a misplaced trust, as no book of this nature can be sufficiently comprehensive in its content. It is hoped that readers will find this book a useful adjunct to broad based reading in Radiology while helping their preparation for the examination itself.

We are indebted to Miss Joan Doyle for her help in preparing the manuscript. Finally we wish to thank our wives, Chris and Jackie, for their patience and encouragement.

Richard Mendelson                                         Graham Whitehouse

# Questions

# Gastrointestinal Tract and Adnexa

Q1  Causes of dysphagia include:
    a  cytomegalovirus infection
    b  varices
    c  African Trypanosomiasis
    d  epidermolysis bullosa
    e  polymyalgia rheumatica

Q2  The following statements are true of post-cricoid web:
    a  they are easily demonstrated by endoscopy
    b  they usually occur on the posterior wall of the hypopharynx
    c  there is an association with intestinal malabsorption
    d  there is an increased risk of carcinoma
    e  there is an association with pernicious anaemia

Q3  The following are recognized radiological signs of reflux oesophagitis:
    a  diffuse granular mucosal pattern
    b  transverse striations
    c  intramural pseudodiverticulosis
    d  reticular mucosal pattern
    e  pulsion diverticulum

Q4  The following are true of Barrett's oesophagus
    a  squamous carcinoma of the oesophagus is a complication
    b  there is a congenitally short oesophagus in most patients
    c  ulcers only occur at or above the squamo-columnar junction
    d  gastro-oesophageal reflux is almost universally present
    e  the distal oesophagus may show a reticular pattern on double contrast swallow

Q5  The following statements are true of oesophageal carcinoma:
    a  most are adenocarcinomas
    b  computed tomography is accurate in assessing tumour resectability
    c  there is an association with gastro-oesophageal reflux
    d  there is an association with asbestos exposure
    e  there is an association with ulcerative colitis

**Q6** Oesophagogastroduodenoscopy is superior to double contrast barium meal in the diagnosis of:
   a  intramural pseudodiverticulosis of the oesophagus
   b  cricopharyngeal web
   c  Schatzki ring
   d  erosive gastritis
   e  stomal ulceration after partial gastrectomy

**Q7** In acute upper gastrointestinal bleeding:
   a  acute gastric erosion is the commonest diagnosis in the UK
   b  in patients with oesophageal varices, other lesions are the cause of bleeding in about 50%
   c  the increased use of endoscopy has resulted in a significant reduction in mortality
   d  a visible vessel in an ulcer crater on endoscopy signifies a high risk of recurrent bleeding
   e  Mallory-Weiss syndrome carries a high mortality

**Q8** The following statements are true of gastric polyps:
   a  adenomas are a recognized feature of pernicious anaemia
   b  adenomas are premalignant
   c  adenomas are the commonest polyps
   d  hyperplastic polyps are premalignant
   e  gastric hamartomas are a recognized association in familial adenomatous polyposis of the colon

**Q9** Increased gastric acid secretion is a recognized feature in the following conditions:
   a  Ménétrièr's disease
   b  acute erosive gastritis
   c  vipoma
   d  most patients with gastric ulcer
   e  hyperparathyroidism

**Q10** The H2 receptor antagonists:
   a  inhibit gall bladder emptying
   b  prevent stress ulcers in seriously ill patients
   c  arrest acute bleeding in chronic duodenal ulceration
   d  are of benefit in the treatment of Zollinger-Ellison syndrome
   e  reduce bleeding in the Mallory-Weiss syndrome

Q11 Recognized complications of selective vagotomy include:
a an increased incidence of gall-stones
b lower oesophageal obstruction
c bradycardia
d gastric stasis
e chronic constipation

Q12 Recognized complications of partial gastrectomy include:
a osteomalacia
b cirrhosis
c megaloblastic anaemia
d malignancy in the gastric remnant
e pulmonary tuberculosis

Q13 The following statements are true of congenital pyloric stenosis:
a symptoms are usually present from birth
b it is commoner in males
c ultrasound examination is useful in the diagnosis
d there is an association with Down's syndrome
e there is an association with anal atresia

Q14 Thickened small bowel folds are typically seen in:
a uncomplicated coeliac disease
b intestinal lymphangiectasia
c systemic sclerosis
d primary lactase deficiency
e Crohn's disease

Q15 The following occur predominantly on the mesenteric border of the small intestine:
a Meckel's diverticulum
b ulceration in Crohn's disease
c jejunal diverticulosis
d haematogenous metastases
e pseudosacculation in Crohn's disease

**Q16** The following are causes of small intestine strictures:
a   eosinophilic gastroenteritis
b   non-granulomatous ulcerative jejunitis
c   amyloidosis
d   mastocytosis
e   systemic sclerosis

**Q17** The following are recognized associations:
a   coeliac disease and splenic atrophy
b   Crohn's disease and chronic pancreatitis
c   renal oxalate stones developing after ileal resection for Crohn's disease
d   giardiasis and jejunal stricture
e   Crohn's disease and retroperitoneal fibrosis

**Q18** Complications of coeliac disease include:
a   hypertrophic osteo-arthropathy
b   jejunal ulceration
c   carcinoma of the oesophagus
d   lymphoma
e   primary sclerosing cholangitis

**Q19** The following statements are true:
a   alopecia is associated with colonic polyposis
b   adenomas are present from birth in familial adenomatous polyposis of the colon
c   gastric hamartomas are associated with Peutz-Jegher syndrome
d   carcinoma of the peri-ampullary region is associated with multiple osteomas
e   Peutz-Jegher syndrome most commonly presents with acute gastrointestinal bleeding

**Q20** *Yersinia enterocolitica:*
a   is a fungus
b   may produce colonic aphthoid ulceration
c   causes bowel strictures
d   is a cause of terminal ileitis
e   is a cause of intra-abdominal abscess

## Gastrointestinal Tract and Adnexa 7

**Q21** The following statements are true of intussusception:
  a  it is the commonest cause of an 'acute abdomen' in 1 year olds
  b  rectal bleeding is a contra-indication to attempted reduction by barium enema
  c  has characteristic ultrasonographic appearances
  d  there is an association with Henoch-Schonlein purpura
  e  a predisposing cause is apparent in most infants

**Q22** The following are true of neonatal necrotizing enterocolitis:
  a  it frequently presents with small bowel distension as the earliest sign
  b  intramural gas may occur in the stomach
  c  there is an association with Hirschsprung's disease
  d  fibrous strictures are a recognized complication
  e  it is a cause of gas in the biliary tract

**Q23** Recognized features of ulcerative colitis include:
  a  venous thrombosis
  b  aphthous ulceration in the mouth
  c  pyoderma gangrenosum
  d  gall-stones
  e  duodenal ulcer

**Q24** Pseudomembranous colitis:
  a  is related to *Clostridium difficile* toxin
  b  is confirmed by culture of *C. difficile*
  c  is associated with colonic 'thumb-printing'
  d  is a strong indication for barium enema
  e  usually involves the rectum

**Q25** The following are features of 'cathartic colon':
  a  loss of haustration principally in the left side of the colon
  b  segmental spasm
  c  *Pneumatosis coli*
  d  degeneration of the myenteric plexus
  e  *Melanosis coli*

**Q26** Pseudo-obstruction of the colon is associated with:
  a  marked fluid distension of the bowel
  b  hyperkalaemia
  c  no risk of caecal perforation
  d  myxoedema
  e  cardiac failure

**Q27** The following statements are true of the solitary rectal ulcer syndrome:
a ulcerative colitis is a cause
b there is an association with rectal prolapse
c it usually occurs in elderly females
d polypoid thickening of a valve of Houston may be seen
e it responds to corticosteroids

**Q28** The following are recognized features of the irritable colon syndrome:
a upper abdominal pain
b alternating constipation and diarrhoea
c alteration in small intestinal motility
d *Pneumatosis coli*
e pain on air insufflation during barium enema

**Q29** Gas in the biliary tract is associated with:
a duodenal ulceration
b hepatic artery occlusion
c diabetes mellitus
d endoscopic sphincterotomy
e old age

**Q30** Primary sclerosing cholangitis:
a is due to gall-stones
b is a frequent occurrence in Crohn's disease
c may progress to cirrhosis
d is associated with cholangiocarcinoma
e is associated with retroperitoneal fibrosis

**Q31** In ultrasound examination of the biliary tract:
a the normal common hepatic duct measures up to 10 mm in internal diameter
b the calibre of the common hepatic duct corresponds with the calibre measured at endoscopic cholangiography
c the common hepatic duct usually dilates after cholecystectomy
d a normal calibre common hepatic duct excludes choledocholithiasis
e in common bile duct obstruction the common hepatic duct dilates before the intrahepatic ducts

## Gastrointestinal Tract and Adnexa 9

**Q32** There is a recognized association between gall-stones and:
  a  primary biliary cirrhosis
  b  carcinoma of the gall bladder
  c  Crohn's disease
  d  Dubin-Johnson syndrome
  e  pernicious anaemia

**Q33** The following statements are true of cholestatic jaundice:
  a  urobilinogen is absent from the urine if obstruction is complete
  b  ultrasound examination reliably visualizes common bile duct calculi
  c  serum alkaline phosphatase is elevated
  d  there is a marked increase in serum transaminase
  e  gall bladder distension suggests choledocholithisasis

**Q34** The following statements are true:
  a  duodenal diverticulum is associated with an increased incidence of common bile duct calculi
  b  duodenal diverticulum may be complicated by duodeno-colic fistula
  c  poor gall bladder emptying occurs in coeliac disease
  d  choledochocele and anal atresia are associated
  e  the calibre of the portal vein on ultrasonography is closely associated to the portal venous pressure

**Q35** Ultrasound examination may show specific diagnostic features in the liver in:
  a  Budd-Chiari syndrome
  b  cavernous haemangioma
  c  metastases from carcinoma of the bronchus
  d  diffuse lymphomatous infiltration
  e  amoebic liver abscess

## Q36 The following statements are true:
a non-visualisation of the gall bladder 60 minutes after injection of Tc-HIDA is diagnostic of acute cholecystitis
b thickening of the gall bladder wall on ultrasonography is a specific feature of acute cholecystitis
c marrow uptake of Tc-labelled sulphur colloid is pathognomic of acute hepatic failure
d Tc-HIDA scintigraphy is useful in differentiating neonatal hepatitis from biliary atresia
e Tc-sodium pertechnetate imaging is useful in suspected Meckel's diverticulum

## Q37 Intrahepatic calcification visible on plain radiography occurs in:
a haemochromatosis
b amoebic abscess
c metastases from carcinoma of the colon
d schistosomiasis
e hepatoma

## Q38 The following statements are true of ultrasound examination:
a the normal pancreas is less echogenic than normal liver
b the normal main pancreatic duct is not visualized
c the pancreas shows increasing echogenicity with age
d ultrasound is superior to computed tomography (CT) in acute pancreatitis
e the gastroduodenal artery cannot be visualized

## Q39 In acute pancreatitis:
a dilatation of the duodenum is the commonest abnormality on plain abdominal radiography
b the colon 'cut-off' sign is pathognomonic
c a left pleural effusion indicates a severe attack
d loss of the left psoas margin may occur
e separation of the stomach and transverse colon is a reliable sign

## Q40 Pancreatic calcification is a recognized feature in:
a tuberculosis
b pancreatic cystadenocarcinoma
c cystic fibrosis
d Wilson's disease
e coeliac disease

## Gastrointestinal Tract and Adnexa

**Q41** The following are true of annular pancreas:
a there is an association with Down's syndrome
b there is a recognized association with malrotation of the gut
c there is a recognized association with choledochal cyst
d there is an increased incidence in maternal diabetes
e it may present with acute gastrointestinal bleeding

**Q42** In systemic sclerosis:
a dilatation of the duodenum occurs
b malabsorption is a recognized complication
c strictures of the colon occur
d small bowel intussusception is a recognized feature
e oesophageal involvement is best demonstrated in the erect position

**Q43** The following are contra-indicated:
a Gastrografin in meconium ileus
b barium by mouth in small bowel obstruction
c barium enema in toxic megacolon
d Gastrografin in tracheo-oesophageal fistula
e barium enema within 6 days of rectal biopsy via a rigid sigmoidoscope

**Q44** The following are true of intravenous glucagon in upper gastrointestinal tract investigation:
a it causes gastro-oesophageal reflux
b small bowel transit time is increased
c it is contra-indicated in glaucoma
d it contracts the gall bladder
e phaeochromocytoma is a contra-indication

**Q45** Recognized causes of hypo-albumenaemia include:
a Ménétrièr's disease
b intestinal lymphangiectasia
c Crohn's disease
d Peutz-Jegher syndrome
e myeloma

# Locomotor System

**Q46** Recognized features of gout include:
 a  poorly defined bone erosions
 b  joint space narrowing occurring early in the disease
 c  severe periarticular osteoporosis
 d  hand involvement most severe in the interphalangeal joints
 e  the presence of bone erosions within 1 year of clinical onset

**Q47** Recognized causes of marginal joint erosions include:
 a  sarcoidosis
 b  hyperparathyroidism
 c  polyarteritis nodosa
 d  haemochromatosis
 e  systemic sclerosis

**Q48** Ulnar deviation is a feature of:
 a  Jaccoud's arthritis
 b  systemic lupus erythematosus
 c  juvenile chronic seronegative arthritis
 d  osteoarthrosis
 e  radial nerve injury

**Q49** There is a recognized association of erosive arthropathy in the hands with:
 a  tuberose sclerosis
 b  Sjogren's syndrome
 c  Jaccoud's arthritis
 d  multicentric reticulohistiocytosis
 e  Reiter's disease

**Q50** The following features distinguish erosive seronegative polyarthritides from rheumatoid arthritis:
 a  pronounced periarticular osteoporosis
 b  florid periosteal new bone formation
 c  tenosynovitis
 d  sacroiliitis
 e  the presence of bony ankylosis

**Q51** There is a strong association between HLA-B27 antigen and:
a Reiter's syndrome
b Behcet's disease
c chronic active hepatitis
d rheumatoid arthritis
e spondylo-arthritis associated with ulcerative colitis

**Q52** In arthritis associated with colitis:
a the activity of the spondylitis of ulcerative colitis parallels that of the colitis
b the hips are the most frequent peripheral joints involved in Crohn's disease
c sacro-iliitis may precede the onset of bowel disease
d the peripheral arthritis parallels the activity of the bowel disease
e Reiter's syndrome may follow *Yersinia enterocolitica* infection

**Q53** Ankylosing spondylitis:
a is commoner in women
b has a recognized association with basal pulmonary fibrosis
c has a recognized association with aortic stenosis
d may be complicated by amyloidosis
e may be complicated by atlanto-axial subluxation

**Q54** Bilateral sacro-iliitis is a recognized feature of:
a intestinal lipodystrophy (Whipple's disease)
b polymyalgia rheumatica
c coeliac disease
d Forestier's disease (ankylosing vertebral hyperostosis)
e Crohn's disease

**Q55** Calcium hydroxyapatite deposition:
a is associated with acutely painful joints
b is associated with diabetes mellitus
c causes the soft tissue calcification in systematic sclerosis
d is associated with acute bursitis
e is the cause of pseudogout

**Q56** Articular chondrocalcinosis is a recognized feature of:
a Wilson's disease
b hyperphosphatasia
c hypoparathyroidism
d amyloidosis
e phenylketonuria

**Q57** Recognized causes of a widened femoral intercondylar notch include:
a haemophilia
b juvenile seronegative arthropathy
c tuberculous arthritis
d synovioma
e Turner's syndrome

**Q58** Causes of avascular necrosis of the femoral head include:
a acute pancreatitis
b Gaucher's disease
c hyperthyroidism
d homocystinuria
e polyarteritis nodosa

**Q59** Perthe's disease:
a occurs bilaterally in most patients
b is commoner in males
c is commonest at puberty
d is associated with accelerated skeletal maturation
e has a worse prognosis in younger patients

**Q60** In infective spondylitis:
a new bone formation strongly suggests a tuberculous aetiology in caucasians
b there is an association with surgery to the lower urinary tract
c rarefaction of the vertebral end plate is an early feature
d tuberculosis may involve the posterior elements alone
e scalloping of the posterior surfaces of the vertebral bodies is a recognized feature

**Q61** Concerning chordoma:
a they mostly occur in young adults
b lung metastases are common
c calcification within the lesion is rare
d the cervical spine is the commonest site
e it may involve two or more adjacent vertebrae

## Locomotor System

**Q62** The following statements are true:
a histiocytosis X is the commonest cause of vertebra plana in adolescence
b the sacrum is the commonest site of giant cell tumour in the spine
c osteoid osteoma of the spine is nearly always located in the vertebral body
d aneurysmal bone cysts do not occur in the spine
e the spine is the commonest site of benign osteoblastomas

**Q63** Posterior scalloping of the vertebral bodies occurs in:
a arachnoid diverticula
b acromegaly
c neurofibromatosis
d long-standing communicating hydrocephalus
e extramedullary haemopoiesis

**Q64** Atlanto-axial subluxation is associated with:
a rheumatoid disease
b ankylosing spondylitis
c Marfan's syndrome
d systemic sclerosis
e ankylosing vertebral hyperostosis

**Q65** In fibrous dysplasia:
a primary malignant bone tumours are a recognized complication
b coarse intraosseous calcification tends to occur with increasing age
c polyostotic disease is usually unilateral
d the condition is much more common in females
e café au lait spots are a recognized association

**Q66** Features of Marfan's syndrome include:
a aortic incompetence
b mental retardation
c osteoporosis
d joint hypermobility
e scoliosis

# Questions

**Q67** Recognized features of thalassaemia major include:
a gram-negative osteomyelitis
b bone infarcts
c narrowing of the foramen magnum
d hypertelorism
e paravertebral soft tissue swelling

**Q68** Recognized features of neurofibromatosis include:
a bone sclerosis
b pseudo-arthrosis
c calverial thickening
d narrowing of the interpedicular distance in the spine
e osteomalacia

**Q69** A small acetabular angle occurs in:
a Morquio-Brailsford disease
b achondroplasia
c congenital hypothyroidism
d Down's syndrome
e Turner's syndrome

**Q70** There is a recognized association of carpal coalition and:
a cleidocranial dysostosis
b Ellis-von Crefeld syndrome
c achondroplasia
d Apert's syndrome
e congenital hypothyroidism

**Q71** The following are recognized associations:
a spinal stenosis and achondroplasia
b colonic polyposis and osteomas of the mandible
c carpal fusion and flat acetabular angles
d carotid artery aneurysms and metacarpal index of 9.5
e multiple naevoid basal cell carcinomas and odontogenic cysts

**Q72** Expansile metastases to bone occur in:
a carcinoma of colon
b carcinoid tumour
c phaeochromocytoma
d transitional cell carcinoma of kidney
e thyroid carcinoma

## Locomotor System

**Q73** Osteoblastic deposits occur in:
a non-Hodgkin's lymphoma
b thyroid papillary carcinoma
c medulloblastoma
d carcinoid tumour
e mucinous carcinoma of the colon

**Q74** The following statements are true:
a calcification occurs frequently in chondromyxoid fibroma
b chondroblastoma presents most often below the age of 10 years
c calcification occurs in benign osteoblastoma in about half the cases
d benign chondroblastoma arises from the epiphysis
e the proximal humerus is the commonest site for fibrous cortical defects

**Q75** Osteoid osteoma:
a rarely occurs in the spine
b is commonest in the 30 to 40 year age group
c is usually located in the epiphysis
d produces a photon-abundant area on bone scintigraphy
e causes pain typically relieved by aspirin

**Q76** The following statements are true:
a the hand is the commonest site of enchondromas
b there is a recognized association between diaphyseal aclasis and haemangiomas
c in dyschondroplasia (Ollier's disease) disparity of limb length is a recognized feature
d chondrosarcoma is the commonest primary malignant tumour of the bony pelvis
e degeneration to osteosarcoma is a frequent complication of diaphyseal aclasis

**Q77** Likely causes of a lesion crossing the epiphyseal growth plate include:
a tuberculosis
b enchondroma
c unicameral bone cyst
d osteosarcoma
e giant cell tumour

**Q78** In multiple myeloma:
  a  bone lesions heal with sclerosis following chemotherapy
  b  spinal cord compression does not occur in the absence of vertebral body collapse
  c  expanding lesions are commoner in long bones than flat bones
  d  radionuclide bone imaging is useful in determining the extent of disease
  e  destruction of the vertebral pedicles is a common finding

**Q79** In osteoclastomas (giant cell tumour):
  a  the region of the knee is the most common site
  b  symmetrical cortical expansion is typical
  c  bone biopsy gives a reliable indication of prognosis
  d  lamellar periosteal reaction is a characteristic feature
  e  soft tissue extension is a reliable indicator of malignancy

**Q80** The following statements are true of osteosarcoma:
  a  parosteal sarcoma most commonly presents in the second decade
  b  computed tomography accurately assesses intramedullary extension of osteosarcoma
  c  pulmonary metastases may be demonstrated on radionuclide bone scintigraphy
  d  metastases occur to bone
  e  pulmonary metastases from parosteal sarcoma are often detectable at the time of presentation

**Q81** The following statements are true:
  a  hypercalcaemia is usually present in renal osteodystrophy
  b  hyperphosphaturia is a cause of rickets
  c  calcium pyrophosphate deposition is the usual aetiology of calcific tendinitis
  d  hyperphosphataemia is seen in primary hyperparathyroidism
  e  there is an association between calcium pyrophosphate deposition disease and hyperparathyroidism

**Q82** The following are associated with hypercalcaemia:
  a  chronic phenytoin ingestion
  b  squamous carcinoma of the bronchus
  c  myxoedema
  d  prolonged immobilization
  e  Cushing's syndrome

## Locomotor System

**Q83** Osteomalacia or rickets may be associated with:
 a phenobarbitone therapy
 b biliary atresia
 c fibrous dysplasia
 d uretero-ileostomy
 e medullary carcinoma of the thyroid

**Q84** Generalized osteoporosis is associated with:
 a excess unmineralized osteoid
 b Turner's syndrome
 c acromegaly
 d primary biliary cirrhosis
 e myxoedema

**Q85** In radionuclide bone imaging:
 a imaging is optimally performed at 1 hour after Tc-polyphosphonate injection.
 b vertebral collapse due to osteoporosis and metastasis is reliably differentiated
 c hypertrophic osteo-arthropathy has a characteristic appearance
 d primary breast carcinoma may accumulate the isotope
 e there is an increased uptake in joints involved with active rheumatoid disease

**Q86** Behcet's disease is associated with:
 a arterial thrombosis
 b an erosive peripheral arthritis in most patients
 c an enthesopathy
 d pulmonary hypertension
 e an ulcerative colitis in the majority of patients

**Q87** Paget's disease of bone:
 a most commonly involves the skull
 b causes incremental fractures on the concave aspect of long bones
 c is associated with increased meningeal vascular grooves
 d is associated with ureteric colic
 e is commoner in Negroes than Europeans

Q88 There is a recognized association between:
a pectus excavatum and rickets
b slipped femoral epiphysis and renal osteodystrophy
c Perthe's disease and congenital dislocation of the hip
d sacral agenesis and maternal diabetes
e protrusio acetabulae and Marfan's syndrome

Q89 Radiolucent transverse metaphyseal bands occur:
a as a normal variant
b in scurvy
c in rickets
d in leukaemia
e in congenital rubella

Q90 Generalized increase in bone density may be associated with:
a arachnodactyly
b splenomegaly
c blue sclera
d otosclerosis
e a monostotic hallux

Q91 Local acceleration of skeletal maturation occurs in association with:
a juvenile seronegative arthropathy
b tuberculosis
c chondroblastoma
d haemophilia
e synovioma

Q92 Rib destruction with an associated soft tissue mass is a recognized feature of:
a myeloma
b non-Hodgkin's lymphoma
c thyroid carcinoma metastasis
d necrotizing pulmonary aspergillosis
e actinomycosis

Q93 Recognized causes of pseudarthrosis include:
a osteogenesis imperfecta
b Paget's disease
c fibrous dysplasia
d osteopetrosis
e scurvy

**Q94** Soft tissue calcification is a recognized association of:
  a hyperphosphataemia
  b hypoparathyroidism
  c homocystinuria
  d hyperthyroidism
  e pseudoxanthoma elasticum

**Q95** The heel pad is thickened in:
  a phenytoin therapy
  b acromegaly
  c obesity
  d myxoedema
  e plantar fasciitis

# Genitourinary Tract

**Q96** Causes of renal medullary calcification include:
   a  hyperparathyroidism
   b  chronic glomerulonephritis
   c  transplant rejection
   d  renal papillary necrosis
   e  medullary sponge kidney

**Q97** Nephrocalcinosis occurs in:
   a  primary oxaluria
   b  hyperphosphaturic rickets
   c  diabetes insipidus
   d  prolonged bismuth antacid ingestion
   e  hyperthyroidism

**Q98** This and the following two questions are linked.

A 35 year old black female patient is admitted complaining of vomiting for several days. Investigations reveal a blood urea level of 10 times normal, and haemoglobin of 7 grams %. Which of the following diagnoses would you consider likely?

   a  chronic pyelonephritis
   b  acute tubular necrosis
   c  gastroenteritis
   d  bladder outflow obstruction
   e  renal papillary necrosis

**Q99** Which of the following investigations are important in the initial work-up of this patient:
   a  ultrasound examination of the kidneys
   b  radiograph of the hands
   c  micturating cystogram
   d  barium meal
   e  chest radiography

# Genitourinary Tract

Q100  A high-dose intravenous urogram shows small kidneys with papillary deformity and uneven parenchymal thinning. Likely diagnoses include:
- a  chronic glomerulonephritis
- b  chronic pyelonephritis
- c  renal papillary necrosis
- d  post-obstructive atrophy
- e  bilateral renal artery fibromuscular hyperplasia

Q101  Renal papillary necrosis:
- a  is commonest in males
- b  may present with bilateral obstructive uropathy
- c  occurs only in adults
- d  is seen in chronic transplant rejection
- e  is seen in spherocytosis

Q102  The following statements are true of duplex kidneys:
- a  the upper renal moiety ureter terminates below and medial to the lower renal moiety ureter
- b  the upper renal moiety is more prone to obstruction
- c  there is a higher incidence of multiple renal arteries
- d  there is an association with retrocaval ureter
- e  there is an association with medullary sponge kidney

Q103  The following are true of renal vein thrombosis:
- a  ultrasonography is useful in the diagnosis
- b  ureteral notching is a recognized feature
- c  a persistent nephrogram is a recognized feature
- d  there is a recognized association with renal artery fibromuscular hyperplasia
- e  there is an association with sickle cell disease

Q104  Recognized associations of renal calculi include:
- a  corticosteroid therapy
- b  ulcerative colitis
- c  Paget's disease
- d  jejunal bypass surgery
- e  partial gastrectomy

Q105 The following are recognized features of renal cell carcinoma:
a cholestatic jaundice
b seeding of metastases to the bladder
c association with analgesic abuse
d arteriography is as accurate as CT in tumour staging
e there is an increased incidence in horse-shoe kidney

Q106 The following are recognized associations:
a polycystic kidneys and berry aneurysms
b neurofibromatosis and renal artery stenosis
c Wilm's tumour and hemihypertrophy
d polycystic kidneys and biliary atresia
e renal hamartomas and neurofibromatosis

Q107 The following features favour the diagnosis of neuroblastoma over Wilm's tumour:
a calcification
b loss of renal function on the affected side
c extension across the midline
d associated aniridia
e pulmonary metastases

Q108 The following statements are true of transitional cell carcinoma of the renal pelvis:
a there is a recognized association with chronic analgesic ingestion
b calcification is a recognized feature
c they are typically hypervascular in the later arterial phase of renal angiography
d there is a higher incidence in the horse-shoe kidney anomaly
e there is an association with carcinoma of the bladder

Q109 The following are recognized features of a right peri-renal abscess:
a anterior displacement of the descending duodenum
b loss of definition of the inferior angle of the liver
c loss of definition of the properitoneal fat line
d lumbar scoliosis concave to the left
e preservation of the psoas outline

Genitourinary Tract

Q110 The following are causes of a unilateral large kidney:
 a xanthogranulomatous pyelonephritis
 b acute pyelonephritis
 c multicystic kidney
 d adult polycystic disease
 e acute glomerulonephritis

Q111 Cysts within the kidney occur in:
 a long-term haemodialysis
 b tuberose sclerosis
 c Turner's syndrome
 d fibrocystic disease of the pancreas
 e Von Hippel-Lindau syndrome

Q112 The following statements are true of the horse-shoe kidney anomaly:
 a There is a recognized association with abdominal aortic aneurysm
 b there is an increased incidence of renal cell carcinoma
 c there is an increased incidence of nephroblastoma
 d the isthmus consists of fibrous tissue in the majority
 e upper urinary tract obstruction is more common on the right side

Q113 Nephrotic syndrome has a recognised association with:
 a sarcoidosis
 b lymphoma
 c Nail-patella (Fong's) syndrome
 d systemic lupus erythematosus
 e Gaucher's disease

Q114 In medullary sponge kidney:
 a renal function is usually normal
 b there is an association with hepatic fibrosis
 c presentation is usually in childhood
 d there is an overall increase in renal size
 e haematuria is a presenting feature

Q115 In xanthogranulomatous pyelonephritis:
a the erythrocyte sedimentation rate is typically normal
b there is a higher incidence in children than in adults
c neovascularity is a recognized feature on renal angiography
d there is often extension into the perinephric tissues
e urinary calculi are usually present

Q116 Recognized associations of vesico-ureteric reflux include:
a ectopic ureter
b cystitis
c prune-belly syndrome
d retroperitoneal fibrosis
e medullary sponge kidney

Q117 Retroperitoneal fibrosis:
a is typically associated with elevation of erythrocyte sedimentation rate
b is associated with beta-blocking drugs
c has a recognized association with carcinoid tumour
d causes medial deviation of the ureters in the vast majority of cases
e causes obliteration of the psoas outlines early in the disease

Q118 Lateral compression of the bladder is caused by:
a inferior vena cava obstruction
b pelvic lipomatosis
c retroperitoneal fibrosis
d endometriosis
e neurofibromatosis

Q119 Bladder wall calcification is a recognized feature of:
a schistosomiasis
b alkaline cystitis
c malacoplakia
d oxaluria
e lymphogranuloma venereum

## Genitourinary Tract

Q120 **A medial situation of both ureters occurs:**
  a following abdomino-perineal resection
  b in pelvic lipomatosis
  c in West Indian males as a normal variant
  d in prune-belly syndrome
  e during pregnancy

Q121 **Oligohydramnios is associated with:**
  a renal agenesis
  b post-maturity
  c maternal gestation diabetes
  d osteogenesis imperfecta
  e oesophageal atresia

Q122 **The following statements are true of obstetric ultrasound examination:**
  a spina bifida is reliably diagnosed at 14 weeks gestation
  b there is a recognized association between single umbilical artery and fetal anomaly
  c the diagnosis of duodenal obstruction cannot be established by antenatal ultrasound
  d most cases of anencephaly are associated with polyhydramnios
  e calcification in the placenta is associated with intra-uterine growth retardation

Q123 **In obstetric ultrasound examination the following are true:**
  a the fetal heart can be reliably detected at 6 weeks gestation
  b biparietal diameter is an accurate measurement of gestational age up to 36 weeks
  c fetal growth retardation affects abdominal perimeter before biparietal diameter
  d placenta previa may be falsely diagnosed in the presence of an overdistended maternal bladder
  e an enlarged placenta is a feature of maternal diabetes mellitus

**Q124** The following are recognized associations:
  a  ovarian fibroma and pleural effusion
  b  hydatidiform mole and theca lutein cysts
  c  intermittent hydronephrosis and endometriosis
  d  benign cystic teratoma of the ovary (dermoid cyst) and von Hippel Lindau syndrome
  e  myxoedema and carcinoma of the body of the uterus

**Q125** The following statements are true:
  a  delineation of crypts in the uterine wall on hysterosalpingography is pathognomonic of adenomyosis
  b  there is an association between unicornuate uterus and ipsilateral absent kidney
  c  the second half of the menstrual cycle is the optimum time to perform hysterosalpingography
  d  diverticulosis of the fallopian tubes is a manifestation of tuberculosis salpingitis
  e  fallopian tubes calcification is a recognized feature of diabetes mellitus

**Q126** The following are recognized associations:
  a  pneumoperitoneum and bladder prolapse
  b  masculinization and ovarian dermoid cysts
  c  hirsutism and polycystic ovaries
  d  uterine arteriovenous fistula and treated chorio-carcinoma
  e  hysterectomy and postoperative ureteric stricture

# Respiratory System

Q127 **The following statements are true of emphysema:**
  a  panacinar emphysema is seen in non-smokers
  b  centrilobular emphysema usually co-exists with chronic bronchitis
  c  centrilobular emphysema predominantly affects the lower lung zones
  d  panacinar emphysema patients tend to have central cyanosis
  e  centrilobular emphysema rarely leads to cor pulmonale

Q128 **Alpha-1 antitrypsin deficiency is associated with:**
  a  emphysema
  b  hilar lymphadenopathy
  c  cirrhosis
  d  pancreatic neoplasms
  e  gall-stones

Q129 **The following are recognized features of cystic fibrosis:**
  a  chronic pancreatitis
  b  hypertrophic pulmonary osteo-arthropathy
  c  rectal prolapse
  d  neonatal hyaline membrane disease
  e  pneumatosis intestinalis

Q130 **There is a recognized association between bronchiectasis and:**
  a  sequestrated pulmonary segment
  b  agammaglobulinaemia
  c  congenital pulmonary artery hypoplasia
  d  Wegener's granulomatosis
  e  whooping cough

## Q131 The following statements are true of sarcoidosis:
a erythema nodosum is strongly associated with bilateral hilar lymphadenopathy
b pulmonary parenchymal involvement completely resolves in the majority of patients
c pleural effusion does not occur
d anterior mediastinal lymph nodes are usually involved in the presence of hilar lymph node enlargement
e pulmonary fibrosis typically occurs in the lower lobes

## Q132 The following statements are true of Macleod's syndrome:
a the cause is a congenital anomaly of the bronchi
b an expiratory chest film shows air-trapping
c pulmonary angiography is normal
d the abnormality may affect only one lobe
e bronchography demonstrates dilatation of segmental bronchi

## Q133 The following are recognized associations
a narcotic analgesics and pulmonary oedema
b duanorubicin (Adriamycin) and pulmonary fibrosis
c hydralazine and pleural effusion
d chlorpromazine and interstitial pulmonary fibrosis
e phenytoin and hilar enlargement

## Q134 The following statements are true:
a in Bird Fancier's Lung there is predominantly upper lobe involvement in the acute phase
b pleural effusion is common in Bird Fancier's Lung
c bronchial wall thickening is the commonest radiological abnormality in allergic bronchopulmonary aspergillosis
d immunosuppressed patients are at risk of developing allergic bronchopulmonary aspergillosis
e exposure to epoxy resin may result in eosinophilic pneumonia

# Respiratory System

**Q135** Blood eosinophilia and pulmonary opacities are associated in:
- a ascariasis
- b sarcoid
- c Churg-Strauss syndrome
- d Hodgkin's disease
- e salicylate ingestion

**Q136** The following statements are true:
- a berylliosis causes bilateral hilar lymph node enlargement
- b talc exposure predisposes to malignant mesothelioma
- c emphysema is the predominant radiological feature of chronic cadmium intoxication
- d the main radiological feature of byssinosis is pulmonary fibrosis
- e carbon monoxide inhalation causes pulmonary oedema

**Q137** The following are true of asbestos exposure:
- a Caplan's syndrome does not occur in asbestosis
- b asbestos exposure predisposes to gastric carcinoma
- c pleural effusion in asbestos exposure invariably indicates mesothelioma
- d there is a predisposition to tuberculosis
- e parenchymal involvement of the lung does not occur without pleural involvement

**Q138** Recognized features of silicosis include:
- a discrete nodules are predominantly basal
- b lymph node calcification is seen
- c calcification of pulmonary nodules may occur
- d cavitation occurs only in the presence of tuberculosis
- e conglomerate lesions are typically in the apical segments of the lower lobes

**Q139** In pneumocystis pneumonia:
- a the diagnosis is established by an increase in specific serum precipitin levels
- b there is predominantly upper lobe involvement
- c cavitation is frequent
- d Septrin (cotrimoxazole) is the drug of first choice
- e septal lines are a recognized feature

Q140 Concerning bronchogenic neoplasms the following are true:
 a the commonest variety is oat-cell carcinoma
 b adenocarcinoma is usually hilar in location
 c there is an association of adenocarcinoma with interstitial pulmonary fibrosis
 d hypertrophic pulmonary osteoarthropathy is more common in oat-cell carcinoma than in other cell types
 e phrenic nerve palsy indicates inoperability

Q141 Bronchial adenomas:
 a are of low-grade malignancy
 b typically occur in elderly patients
 c are best removed endoscopically
 d occur mostly in the perihilar region
 e may cause bronchiectasis

Q142 Recognized features of bronchio-alveolar carcinoma include:
 a frequent occurrence of cavitation in larger lesions
 b association with pleural retraction
 c air bronchograms within the tumour
 d a solitary pulmonary nodule
 e rare occurrence of extrathoracic metastases

Q143 The following statements are true of lung involvement with lymphoma:
 a it is commoner in non-Hodgkin's lymphoma than in Hodgkin's lymphoma at the time of presentation
 b mediastinal lymph node enlargement is usually present
 c solitary lobar consolidation is a recognized manifestation
 d cavitation indicates concurrent infection
 e pulmonary collapse is usually due to bronchial compression by lymph nodes

Q144 There is a recognized association between bronchial carcinoma and:
 a nickel refining
 b Dupuytren's contracture
 c acanthosis nigricans
 d furniture manufacture
 e hyperaldosteronism

Respiratory System 33

Q145 **Likely causes of lymphangitis carcinomatosa include:**
a pancreatic carcinoma
b carcinoma of the colon
c hepatoma
d carcinoma of the cervix
e carcinoma of oesophagus

Q146 **Kerley B lines may be seen as a feature of:**
a bronchopneumonia
b tricuspid incompetence
c lymphoma
d pulmonary haemosiderosis
e sarcoid

Q147 **Causes of pulmonary arterial hypertension include:**
a choriocarcinoma
b secundum atrial septal defect
c carcinoid syndrome
d kyphoscoliosis
e schistosomiasis

Q148 **The following statements are true of radionuclide lung imaging:**
a a hilar carcinoma may cause a ventilation defect with a normal perfusion study
b matched perfusion/ventilation defects may be seen in acute asthma
c perfusion imaging is best performed with the patient supine
d a normal perfusion study virtually excludes pulmonary embolism
e left lower lobe perfusion is often reduced in cardiomegaly

Q149 **Pulmonary oedema with a normal-sized heart occurs in:**
a acute glomerulonephritis
b myocardial infarction
c brainstem haemorrhage
d acute rupture of chordae tendinae
e hypertrophic obstructive cardiomyopathy

Q150 Causes of unilateral left-sided pulmonary oedema include:
a right-sided Blalock-Taussig anastomosis
b left pulmonary vein occlusion
c rapid thoracentesis of a large left pleural effusion
d massive left-sided pulmonary embolus
e left-sided pulmonary contusion

Q151 Enlargement of the azygos vein occurs in:
a pregnancy
b thymic tumours
c portal hypertension
d inferior vena cava obstruction
e superior vena cava obstruction

Q152 The following are recognized associations:
a transient tachypnoea of the newborn and elective Caesarian section
b pulmonary hypoplasia and renal agenesis
c neonatal pneumothorax and biliary atresia
d tracheo-oesophageal fistula and maternal diabetes
e hyaline membrane disease and maternal diabetes

Q153 The following are recognized features of meconium aspiration:
a an association with post-maturity
b areas of hyperinflation are common
c bronchopulmonary dysplasia is the usual sequel in survivors
d patients are usually suffering from fibrocystic disease
e pneumomediastinum is a recognized complication

Q154 The following are true of intralobar pulmonary sequestration:
a the arterial supply is from a pulmonary artery
b the venous drainage is usually to the inferior vena cava
c it is most commonly right-sided
d it may present with haemoptysis
e it may cavitate

# Respiratory System

Q155 **Pulmonary cavitation is a recognized feature of:**
   a pulmonary contusion
   b pulmonary infarction
   c Wegener's granuloma
   d osteosarcoma metastases
   e adult respiratory distress syndrome

Q156 **Pulmonary calcification is a recognized feature of:**
   a toxoplasmosis
   b psittacosis
   c varicella pneumonia
   d renal failure
   e asbestosis

Q157 **The following statements are true of pulmonary hamartomas:**
   a calcification is seen in most cases
   b fat may be demonstrated on CT within the lesion
   c cavitation does not occur
   d they increase in size after childhood
   e the majority of cases are discovered over the age of 40 years

Q158 **Causes of pneumothorax include:**
   a endometriosis
   b diabetic ketoacidosis
   c osteosarcoma metastases
   d osteochondroma of the ribs
   e hamartoma of the lung

Q159 **Enlarged paratracheal lymph nodes are a recognized radiographic feature of:**
   a post-primary tuberculosis
   b Legionnaire's disease
   c extramedullary haemopoiesis
   d infectious mononucleosis
   e Wegener's granulomatosis

**Q160 Thymic enlargement:**
   a  occurs in the majority of patients with myasthenia gravis
   b  is a cause of dysphagia
   c  is more prominent in inspiration in infants
   d  occurs in severe infection in infancy
   e  is associated with thyrotoxicosis

**Q161 Fracture of a bronchus:**
   a  is associated with fracture of the upper ribs
   b  is invariably associated with pneumothorax
   c  is commoner on the left
   d  usually involves an intrapulmonary bronchus
   e  may present as delayed bronchial stenosis

# Cardiovascular System

Q162 The following are recognized associations:
  a  pulmonary stenosis and Noonan's syndrome
  b  supravalvar aortic stenosis and Turner's syndrome
  c  primum atrial septal defect and heart block
  d  Marfan's syndrome and aortic stenosis
  e  hypercalcaemia and peripheral pulmonary artery stenosis

Q163 Coarctation of the aorta is associated with:
  a  rib notching which usually appears during infancy
  b  intracranial aneurysms
  c  Fallot's tetralogy
  d  aortic stenosis
  e  left ventricular failure during the neonatal period

Q164 The following are recognized associations:
  a  total anomalous pulmonary venous drainage and polysplenia
  b  peripheral pulmonary artery stenoses and maternal hypothyroidism
  c  right-sided aortic arch and ventricular septal defect
  d  pulmonary artery calcification and atrial septal defect
  e  supravalvar aortic stenosis and hypercalcaemia

Q165 **The following cause neonatal cyanosis with pulmonary plethora:**
  a  Ebstein's anomaly
  b  total anomalous pulmonary venous drainage
  c  transposition of the great vessels
  d  truncus arteriosus
  e  anomalous origin of the left coronary artery

**Q166** The following are recognized features of secundum type of atrial septal defect:
a prominent aortic arch
b prominence of the left atrial appendage
c right-sided aortic arch
d enlarged right atrium
e enlarged right ventricle

**Q167** The following statements are true:
a aneurysms of the sinus of Valsalva sometimes rupture into the right ventricle
b post-stenotic dilatation of the pulmonary artery is a recognized feature of Fallot's tetralogy
c pulmonary venous hypertension occurs in left atrial myxoma
d pulmonary artery hypertension is a recognized feature of carcinoid syndrome
e congenital hypertrophic obstructive cardiomyopathy is a recognized occurrence in maternal diabetes

**Q168** The following statements are true of patent ductus arteriosus:
a the aortic arch is usually small
b premature infants are prone to delayed closure
c enlargement of the heart in hyaline membrane disease suggests the diagnosis
d ultrasound examination is of little value in establishing the diagnosis in neonates
e calcification of the ductus occurs in long-standing cases

**Q169** There is a recognized association between cardiomyopathy and:
a biliary cirrhosis
b Friedrich's ataxia
c Addison's disease
d sarcoid
e pernicious anaemia

## Cardiovascular System 39

**Q170** The following are recognized associations
  a atrial septal defect and absent thumbs
  b coarctation of the aorta and bronchial carcinoid
  c joint hypermobility and mitral incompetence
  d sarcoidosis and complete heart block
  e Raynaud's disease and aortic stenosis

**Q171** Post-myocardial infarction (Dressler's) syndrome:
  a usually occurs within 24 hours of myocardial infarction
  b responds to corticosteroids
  c is associated with pleural effusion
  d is accompanied by a normal erythrocyte sedimentation rate
  e the echocardiogram is usually normal

**Q172** There is a recognized association between mitral valve prolapse and:
  a Marfan's syndrome
  b pectus excavatum
  c thoracic scoliosis
  d secundum atrial septal defect
  e ankylosing spondylitis

**Q173** Central cyanosis is a feature of:
  a chronic obstructive airways disease
  b right to left intracardiac shunt
  c severe anaemia with cardiac failure
  d carbon monoxide poisoning
  e Fallot's tetralogy

**Q174** The following statements are true of radionuclide cardiac imaging:
  a Thallium-$^{201}$ imaging demonstrates ischaemic myocardium as a 'hot-spot'
  b increased uptake of Tc-pyrophosphate by myocardium is specific for acute myocardial infarction
  c maximal sensitivity for Tc-pyrophosphate imaging in myocardial infarction occurs at 24 hours after infarction
  d the prognosis is worse if pyrophosphate imaging is persistently positive after myocardial infarction
  e thallium imaging can distinguish between infarcted myocardium and ischaemic but viable myocardium

**Q175** Causes of left ventricular enlargement include:
  a  pure mitral stenosis
  b  tricuspid atresia
  c  anomalous left coronary artery
  d  Ebstein's anomaly
  e  truncus arteriosus

**Q176** The following statements are true of pericardial effusion:
  a  uraemia is a cause
  b  pulmonary congestion is typical
  c  the heart borders are poorly defined
  d  there is absence of the pericardial fat line on lateral radiographs
  e  the posterior convexity of the cardiac shadow is markedly accentuated on lateral radiographs

**Q177** The following statements are true of thoracic aortic dissection:
  a  displacement of the left main bronchus is a recognized feature on plain chest radiography
  b  computed tomography is highly accurate in detecting the site of the intimal tear
  c  computed tomography accurately predicts coronary artery involvement in proximal dissections
  d  a normal echocardiogram is highly accurate in excluding a proximal dissection
  e  medial displacement of intimal calcification in the aortic arch is a specific change on chest radiography

**Q178** Micro-aneurysms of the intrarenal arteries occur in:
  a  polyarteritis nodosa
  b  drug abusers
  c  Takayashu's disease
  d  polymyalgia rheumatica
  e  chronic glomerulonephritis

**Q179** The following are true of traumatic rupture of the thoracic aorta:
  a  the left main bronchus is displaced posteriorly
  b  there is widening of the right paratracheal line
  c  most occur just distal to the aortic valve
  d  most patients who survive the immediate trauma can be managed conservatively
  e  a left apical pleural cap is an early sign

Q180 Mycotic aneurysms:
- a rarely rupture
- b thrombose frequently
- c frequently calcify
- d may be caused by contiguous spread from adjacent infection
- e are commonly sited in the renal arteries

Q181 Arterial calcification is a recognized feature of:
- a homocystinuria
- b Marfan's syndrome
- c calcium pyrophosphate deposition disease
- d Takayasu's arteritis
- e pseudoxanthoma elasticum

# Central Nervous System and Skull

Q182 Basal ganglia calcification occurs in:
  a  congenital toxoplasmosis
  b  radiotherapy to the head
  c  diabetes mellitus
  d  hypoparathyroidism
  e  phenytoin therapy

Q183 Enlargement of the optic canal occurs in:
  a  orbital pseudotumour
  b  Treacher-Collins syndrome
  c  retinoblastoma
  d  craniostenosis
  e  neurofibromatosis

Q184 An enlarged pituitary fossa on plain skull radiography occurs in:
  a  myotonic dystrophy
  b  nearly all patients with craniopharyngioma
  c  most patients with prolactinoma
  d  most patients with Cushing's syndrome
  e  raised intracranial pressure

Q185 Multiple wormian bones are a recognized feature in:
  a  osteogenesis imperfecta
  b  acrocephalosyndactyly (Apert's syndrome)
  c  pseudohypoparathyroidism
  d  cleidocranial dysostosis
  e  chronic raised intracranial pressure

Q186 Calcification in the orbit on plain radiography is a recognized feature of:
  a  retinoblastoma
  b  meningioma of the optic nerve sheath
  c  venous malformation
  d  melanoma
  e  optic nerve glioma

## Central Nervous System and Skull

**Q187** Generalized increase in density of the base of the skull occurs in:
a pyknodysostosis
b phenytoin therapy
c meningioma
d chordoma
e fluorosis

**Q188** The following are recognized causes of parasellar calcification:
a ependymoma
b tuberculous meningitis
c carotico-cavernous sinus fistula
d basilar artery aneurysm
e meningioma

**Q189** The following typically appear as high attenuation lesions on CT in the absence of intravenous contrast injection:
a colloid cyst of the third ventricle
b intracerebral haematoma
c porencephalic cyst
d recent subdural haematoma
e metastasis from bronchial carcinoma

**Q190** Unenhanced magnetic resonance imaging is superior to unenhanced CT in the demonstration of:
a posterior fossa tumours
b demyelinating disease
c intracranial calcification
d subdural haematoma
e meningioma

**Q191** The following lesions typically show marked enhancement with intravenous contrast medium on CT:
a meningioma
b choroid plexus papilloma
c metastasis
d cerebral contusion
e chordoma

## Q192 The following are recognized associations:
a  renal cysts and haemangioblastomas
b  paraventricular calcification and port-wine stain
c  absent zygomatic arch and occlusion of the external auditory meatus
d  chordoma and neurofibromatosis
e  pituitary adenomas and renal hamartomas

## Q193 Causes of Horner's syndrome include:
a  carcinoma of the bronchus
b  syringobulbia
c  subclavian steal syndrome
d  carotid artery aneurysm
e  tertiary syphilis

## Q194 The following statements are true of acoustic neuromas:
a  plain radiography demonstrates widening of the internal auditory meati in the vast majority of patients
b  On CT they are typically hypodense relative to brain
c  there is marked enhancement with intravenous contrast medium on CT
d  CT is superior to magnetic resonance imaging for diagnosis
e  air meatography is often required to augment CT in lesions smaller than 1 cm

## Q195 The following statements are true of subarachnoid haemorrhage:
a  third nerve palsy usually indicates an anterior communicating artery aneurysm
b  intracerebral vascular spasm at angiography is maximal within 3 days of the ictus
c  the demonstration of blood in the subarachnoid space on CT obviates the need for lumbar puncture in suspected subarachnoid haemorrhage
d  it is most commonly due to an aneurysm of the basilar artery
e  there are multiple aneurysms on angiography in about one fifth of patients

**Q196** **The following are true of prolactinomas:**
  a  amenorrhoea is the commonest presenting feature
  b  galactorrhoea is a recognized presenting feature
  c  hypocycloidal tomography will reliably show abnormalities of the sella in more than half the patients
  d  dynamic CT, with intravenous contrast enhancement, will show most prolactinomas to have a higher attenuation than normal pituitary gland
  e  calcification does not occur

# Endocrine System and Metabolism

(See Locomotor System for Metabolic Bone Disease)

**Q197** The features of Cushing's syndrome include:
   a  hyperkalaemia
   b  an adrenal neoplasm in the majority of patients
   c  diabetes mellitus
   d  anaemia
   e  hypocalcaemia

**Q198** The radiological features of Cushing's syndrome include:
   a  exuberant callus in relation to fractures
   b  calcification of the external ear
   c  increased attenuation of the liver on CT
   d  enlargement of the pituitary fossa in most patients
   e  widened mediastinum

**Q199** The following statements are true of phaeochromocytoma:
   a  they are usually malignant
   b  diagnosis is made by an increase in hydroxy-indole acetic acid in the urine
   c  there is a higher proportion of extra-adrenal tumours in children than in adults
   d  they are usually intrathoracic when not adrenal
   e  there is an association with hyperparathyroidism

**Q200** Causes of adrenal calcification include:
   a  amyloid disease
   b  phaeochromocytoma
   c  primary adrenal carcinoma
   d  congenital adrenogenital syndrome
   e  Friderichsen-Waterhouse syndrome

# Endocrine System and Metabolism 47

**Q201** The following statements are true of adrenal imaging:
  a  CT is the primary imaging modality of choice in suspected adrenal disease
  b  $I^{131}$-Metaiodobenzylguanidine is useful in the diagnosis of malignant phaeochromocytoma
  c  Conn's adenoma shows as a 'cold spot' after injection of Se-6-selenomethyl cholesterol (Scintadren)
  d  dexamethasone administration stimulates normal adrenal function
  e  ultrasonography is accurate in the detection of a left adrenal adenoma

**Q202** There is a recognized association between:
  a  thyroid acropachy and pretibial myxoedema
  b  medullary carcinoma of the thyroid and calcified pulmonary metastases
  c  simple colloid goitre and basophil adenoma of the pituitary
  d  medullary carcinoma of the thyroid and megacolon
  e  myxoedema and renal calculi

**Q203** In the investigation of thyroid disease:
  a  thyroid ultrasonography can reliably distinguish benign from malignant nodules
  b  thyroid carcinomas are most often of increased echo-genicity relative to normal thyroid gland on ultrasonography
  c  a cystic component to a nodule suggests benignity
  d  a solitary cold nodule on radionuclide imaging of a multinodular thyroid goitre has a high probability of malignancy
  e  needle biopsy of a solitary thyroid nodule is a highly accurate method in distinguishing benign from malignant disease

**Q204** The following statements are true:
  a  the majority of patients with primary hyperparathyroidism have multiple parathyroid adenomas
  b  there is a direct correlation between the degree of hypercalcaemia and the size of parathyroid tumours
  c  nodular thyroid disease is associated with hyperparathyroidism
  d  high-resolution ultrasonography is of low specificity in the diagnosis of parathyroid adenomas
  e  Thallium $^{201}$ — Technetium $^{99m}$ subtraction scintigraphy is of value in the detection of parathyroid adenomas

Q205 The following statements are true:
- a ectopic ACTH production is most commonly due to squamous carcinoma of the lung
- b hypercalcaemia is a recognized feature of non-metastatic squamous carcinoma of the lung
- c diabetes mellitus is a feature of retroperitoneal sarcoma
- d gynaecomastia is seen in testicular teratoma
- e renal carcinoma is the most frequent origin of inappropriate anti-diuretic hormone

Q206 Gynaecomastia is a feature of:
- a hyperprolactinaemia
- b Klinefelter's syndrome
- c carcinoma of the head of the pancreas
- d cimetidine treatment
- e hyperthyroidism

Q207 The following are recognized associations:
- a peptic ulceration and pancreatic adenoma
- b Zollinger-Ellison syndrome and pituitary adenoma
- c watery diarrhoea and achlorhydria
- d rapid transit of barium through the small bowel and medullary carcinoma of the thyroid
- e increased urinary vanillyl-mandelic acid and achlorhydria

Q208 Causes of hypokalaemia include:
- a Conn's tumour
- b renal tubular acidosis
- c acute tubular necrosis
- d Addison's disease
- e glycosuria

Q209 The following are recognized features of acromegaly:
- a hypertension
- b kyphoscoliosis
- c basilar invagination
- d narrowing of joint spaces early in the disease
- e generalized osteoporosis

## Endocrine System and Metabolism

**Q210** There is a recognized association between diabetes mellitus and:
  a  prostatic calcification
  b  arthritis mutilans
  c  accelerated bone maturation in a child
  d  gastric ileus
  e  renal enlargement

**Q211** The following are recognized causes of hypoglycaemia:
  a  Conn's syndrome
  b  hepatoma
  c  adenocarcinoma of the pancreas
  d  cirrhosis
  e  gastrojejunostomy

# Miscellaneous Topics

Q212 The following statements are true of traumatic rupture of the spleen:
   a the majority of patients have a fracture of a left lower rib
   b anteromedial displacement of the stomach is a recognized feature
   c lateral displacement of the left kidney is a recognized feature
   d CT is a highly accurate method of diagnosis
   e splenectomy is indicated in the presence of a subcapsular haematoma because of the high risk of intraperitoneal rupture

Q213 Calcification of the external ear occurs in:
   a congenital hypothyroidism
   b Addison's disease
   c gout
   d calcium pyrophosphate deposition disease
   e relapsing polychondritis

Q214 Juvenile nasopharyngeal angiofibromas:
   a are distinguishable from large adenoids on plain radiographs
   b cause erosion of the sphenoid bone
   c are poorly enhanced by intravenous contrast medium on CT
   d often calcify
   e are commoner in girls than boys

Q215 The following are recognized associations:
   a patent ductus arteriosus and intracerebral aneurysms
   b Klippel-Feil syndrome and inner ear anomalies
   c congenital hypothyroidism and congenital dislocation of the hip
   d Hirschprung's disease and Down's syndrome
   e anterior spinal meningocele and neurenteric cyst

Miscellaneous 51

Q216 Recognized associations of narcotic drug abuse include:
a pneumocystis pneumonia
b pseudo-obstruction of the colon
c pulmonary fibrosis
d radio-opaque renal calculi
e infective spondylitis

Q217 The following radiographic features favour allergic rather than infective sinusitis:
a swelling of the nasal turbinates
b fluid levels in the sinuses
c scalloped appearance to the mucosal thickening
d a solitary rounded soft tissue mass at the base of a maxillary antrum with mucosal thickening
e involvement of the sphenoid sinus

Q218 Scoliosis is a recognized feature of:
a vertebral osteoid osteoma
b irradiation of the immature spine
c retroperitoneal fibrosis
d acute pancreatitis
e poliomyelitis

Q219 Peripheral curvilinear calcification may be seen on mammography in:
a simple cysts
b haematoma
c fibroadenoma
d fat necrosis
e medullary carcinoma

Q220 Aggregations of irregularly shaped microcalcifications in the breast are a recognized feature of:
a fat necrosis
b sclerosing adenosis
c medullary carcinoma
d cystosarcoma phylloides
e plasma cell mastitis

# Answers and Notes

# Gastrointestinal Tract and Adnexa

**A1** **a** *True* **b** *False* **c** *False* **d** *True* **e** *False*
Specific oesophageal infections that cause dysphagia, usually in immunocompromised patients, include Cytomegalovirus, Herpes simplex virus and Candidiasis. All have similar radiographic appearances (small plaque-like filling defects, or, occasionally a 'cobblestone' pattern or shaggy appearance). Herpes may occasionally be distinguished by discrete, sometimes stellate ulcers separated by normal mucosa.

South American trypanosomiasis (Trypanosoma cruzi; Chagas disease) causes achalasia and hence dysphagia; African Trypanosomiasis does not. The bullous dermatoses, i.e. epidermolysis bullosa, pemphigus and pemphigoid, may produce oesophageal webs progressing to strictures in conjunction with skin disease.

**Causes of dysphagia**

*Luminal narrowing*
**1** *Within lumen.* Bolus obstruction (superimposed on other lesion).
**2** *Within wall.*
(a) Inflammatory/post-inflammatory: peptic stricture/reflux; rarely Crohn's; tuberculosis; Schatzki ring; corrosives/lye; iatrogenic — drugs (e.g. enteric K, tetracycline) — nasogastric (NG) tube; radiotherapy; skin diseases — see above; infections.
(b) Neoplastic: carcinoma; lymphoma — rare, usually non-Hodgkin's lymphoma; leiomyoma/leiomyosarcoma.
(c) Others. e.g. Plummer-Vinson syndrome (crico-pharyngeal web) associated with iron deficiency, including post-gastrectomy and malabsorption states. Postoperative (fundoplication, etc).
**3** *Extrinsic.* Pharyngeal pouch — may be associated with chronic distal obstruction; vascular congenital rings, aortic aneurysm, giant left atrium; mediastinal lymph nodes — lymphoma, secondary; thyroid enlargement.

## Gastrointestinal Tract and Adnexa 55

*Neuromuscular ('pseudodysphagia')*
1 *Cricopharynx.* Bulbar or pseudobulbar palsy, e.g. motor neuron disease; myasthenia gravis; globus hystericus (often psychogenic, but some have gastro-oesophageal reflux)
2 *Oesophagus.* Achalasia; systemic sclerosis (CREST syndrome); exaggerated tertiary contractions (diffuse oesophageal spasm or presbyoesophagus); South American trypanosomiasis (Chagas' disease).

Remember lesions in the stomach (carcinoma of the cardia) and even duodenal obstruction may present predominantly with 'dysphagia'.

**REF: R1**

A2   **a** *False* **b** *False* **c** *True* **d** *True* **e** *False*
*Cricopharyngeal webs* occur on the anterior wall of the hypopharynx, not affecting the posterior wall unless they are circumferential. They may be single or multiple and are best, and often only, seen in lateral barium-distended views. Endoscopy is therapeutic in rupturing the membrane, but the web is not usually seen. Webs must be differentiated from the cricopharyngeal impression formed by the submucosal venous plexus in the same area. The latter is more rounded in profile and changes shape. The clinical significance of webs is variable — they are usually an incidental finding. They rarely occlude enough lumen to produce dysphagia.

*Associations*
Iron-deficiency, including that seen in malabsorption. Skin diseases — epidermolysis bullosa; benign mucous pemphigoid.
  *Plummer-Vinson (Paterson-Kelly) Syndrome*: association of glossitis, mucosal changes in mouth, pharynx and oesophagus, dysphagia and anaemia in middle-aged women. Frequent occurrence of webs, membranes and folds. Validity challenged due to the relative infrequency with which component parts of syndrome occur together. Many patients have no web. Many with webs are not anaemic. There is an increased risk of post-cricoid carcinoma.
  In a series of patients with dysphagia examined with cineradiography, webs were found in 15% — often with co-existant local neuromuscular abnormalities.
**REF: R2**

**A3** **a** *True* **b** *True* **c** *True* **d** *True* **e** *False*

Reflux oesophagitis typically affects the distal third. Hiatus hernia and gastro-oesophageal reflux do not necessarily indicate oesophagitis. However, it is unusual to see oesophagitis in their absence.

*Features of reflux oesophagitis on double contrast barium swallow*
1 *Thickened longitudinal folds* normally should not be visible on maximal distension (>2 cm).
2 *Gastro-oesophageal polyp*, continuous with thickened gastric fold (**REF: R3**).
3 *Mucosal abnormalities*: granularity, erosions, ulceration, nodular/cobblestone mucosa.
4 *Limited distensibility*, due to spasm.
5 *Scarring and strictures*.
6 *Transverse folds*, due to contraction of the longitudinal fibres of the muscular mucosa. Occasionally seen in normals (**REF: R4**).
7 *Intramural pseudodiverticulosis of oesophagus*, see **A6**.
8 *Barrett's oesophagus*, may be associated with a reticular mucosal pattern. See **A4**.
**REF: R5**


**A4** **a** *False* **b** *False* **c** *False* **d** *True* **e** *True*

Barrett's oesophagus is secondary to chronic gastro-oesophageal reflux. Most patients are aged 50–70 years, but all ages can be affected, including children. It denotes a disorder in which there is columnar metaplasia of the oesophagus. The squamocolumnar junction can progressively ascend the oesophagus.
*Complications include:*
(a) Strictures — characteristically in mid-oesophagus at the squamocolumnar junction.
(b) Ulcers in the oesophagus — at the squamocolumnar junction or in columnar epithelium.
(c) Adenocarcinoma of the oesophagus.
In some patients a delicate reticular pattern is seen on D.C. oesophagography in the distal oesophagus, and is said to be specific for Barrett's oesophagus.
**REF: R6, R7**

# Gastrointestinal Tract and Adnexa 57

**A5**    **a** *False*   **b** *False*   **c** *True*   **d** *True*   **e** *False*

The vast majority of *primary oesophageal carcinomas* are of squamous cell type. Adenocarcinomas are usually extensions from primary gastric carcinoma, although oesophageal adenocarcinoma is associated with Barrett's oesophagus and hence gastro-oesophageal reflux. Conditions predisposing to squamous carcinoma include chronic corrosive strictures, achalasia, tylosis, and Plummer-Vinson syndrome (in the postcricoid region). There is an increased incidence in coeliac disease and in asbestos exposure.

Computed tomography has limitations in detecting extra-oesophageal spread into mediastinum and regional lymph nodes. The degree of contact with the aorta, and loss of intervening fat planes between oesophagus and aorta, have been suggested as indicators of resectability, but is not very reliable.

**REF: R8, R9, R10**


**A6**    **a** *False*   **b** *False*   **c** *False*   **d** *True*   **e** *True*

*Intramural pseudodiverticulosis of the oesophagus* is a condition of obscure aetiology, mainly affecting the elderly. Its associations include *Candida* infection (32%), diabetes mellitus (21%), gastro-oesophageal reflux (19%) and alcoholism (15%). Radiology is far more sensitive than endoscopy in the diagnosis, only 20% being identified at oesophago-gastro-duodenoscopy (OGD). The appearances at double contrast oesophagography are of very small flask-like outpouchings of barium, usually uniformly distributed, and stenoses in 90% (anywhere in the oesophagus, but most often upper third) (**REF: R11**).

*Cricopharyngeal webs* are usually missed at OGD. However, the passage of the endoscope may be therapeutic. See **A2**.

Much debate continues with regard to the origin of *Schatzki ring* (lower oesophageal mucosal ring). It is probably part of the spectrum of reflux oesophagitis, occurring at the squamocolumnar junction. The radiographic incidence varies considerably and partly reflects the method used to demonstrate them; they will rarely be seen unless a prone swallow is performed. The presence of dysphagia will depend on the internal calibre of the ring. Those wider than 20 mm are rarely symptomatic, while those under 13 mm usually are. (**REF: R12**).

Superficial mucosal lesions such as *erosive gastritis* are more reliably demonstrated by OGD.

OGD is more accurate in the diagnosis of recurrent *stomal ulceration* following gastric surgery. However, barium radiology is often useful for the clarification of post-operative anatomy, and for assessment of emptying of the gastric remnant. Most stomal ulcers occur within six months of surgery.

A7   a *False*   b *True*   c *False*   d *True*   e *False*
Peptic ulceration is the commonest cause of *acute upper gastrointestinal (GI) bleeding* in the UK (duodenal ulcer and gastric ulcer about equal at 25% each). Gastric erosions account for about 5%. In a large American study, erosions were the single most common cause, perhaps related to the prevalence of alcoholism (also reflected in the high incidence of bleeding varices) and the frequent use of nasogastric aspiration (a NG tube itself can produce mucosal lesion).

Although OGD has provided more accurate diagnosis than barium studies, the overall mortality from acute upper GI bleeding has remained constant over the years at about 10%. However, this reflects the current increased age of presentation, the elderly having a greater mortality from upper GI bleeding. Stigmata of recent haemorrhage in an ulcer, as seen at OGD, include clot or a 'visible vessel' in the base. The rate of continued or recurrent bleeding in patients with a 'visible vessel' is in excess of 50%. OGD can therefore help select patients for careful observation and early surgery. It is this capability, plus the therapeutic potential of OGD itself, and the accuracy of diagnosis, that has led to a minimal role for barium studies.
**REF: R13**

A8   a *True*   b *True*   c *False*   d *False*   e *True*

*Gastric polyps*
1 *Hyperplastic polyps*. Associated with gastritis and pernicious anaemia. Random, often multiple and typically small. *Not* premalignant, but an increased risk of malignancy in the same stomach.
2 *Adenomas*. Rare in stomach. Usually solitary in antrum. Larger than hyperplastic polyps. May be multiple in pernicious anaemia. Liable to malignant change.

3 *Hamartoma.* Associated with Familial Adenomatous Polyposis (FAP). Also seen in Peutz-Jegher's syndrome. Filiform inflammatory polyps may occur in Crohn's disease of stomach.
See also **A19**
**REF: R14, R15**

**A9**   **a** *False*   **b** *False*   **c** *False*   **d** *False*   **e** *True*

*Increased gastric acid secretion*
1  This is found in: some patients with duodenal ulcer. Most patients with gastric ulcer have normal basal and maximal acid outputs; some have low acid levels.
2  Hypergastrinaemia. Excess gastrin causes gastric acid hypersecretion when due to:
(a) Zollinger-Ellison syndrome (Gastrinoma or antral G-cell hyperplasia).
(b) Retained antrum. — *Produces Gastrin*
(c) Chronic renal failure (failure of gastrin clearance).
(d) Hypercalcaemia, especially primary hyperparathyroidism — increased incidence of duodenal ulcer, due either to hypercalcaemia itself or multiple endocrine adenopathy (gastrinoma).
**NB.** Other GI complications of primary hyperparathyroidism: acute and chronic pancreatitis, constipation.

*Ménétrièr's disease* is associated with achlorhydria or hypochlorhydria in the majority of cases. The cardinal clinical feature of the disease is gastric protein loss with hypoalbumenaemia.

*Acute erosive gastritis* is not typically associated with increased acid. The mechanism of damage is probably related to failure of maintenance of the gastric mucosal barrier resulting in back-diffusion of acid and/or interference of mucus production. Causes include: aspirin ingestion (especially when combined with alcohol); other drugs, e.g. non-steroidal anti-inflammatory agents; severe physical stress, e.g. hypovolaemic shock, renal failure, sepsis, severe injury and burns, neurological injury. In most patients with acute gastric erosions no cause is found.

*Vipoma* is a non-insulin secreting islet-cell pancreatic adenoma and one of the group of APUDOMAs (amine precursor uptake and decarboxylation cell tumours). It produces the Verner-Morrison syndrome of watery diarrhoea, hypokalaemia, and achorhydria (WDHA).
**REF: R16**

**A10** a *False* b *True* c *False* d *True* e *False*
There is little evidence that H2 receptor antagonists are of benefit in arresting acute bleeding in peptic ulcers. However, they are probably of benefit in acute gastric erosions. In addition they help prevent erosions in acutely ill patients. Symptomatic benefit may be achieved in Zollinger-Ellison syndrome with high-dose treatment with these drugs. Although the weight of evidence suggests some benefit in reflux oesophagitis, this is not universal experience. It should be noted that ulcerating gastric carcinoma may undergo superficial healing, and the symptoms may be temporarily relieved by Cimetidine or Ranitidine.

**A11** a *False* b *True* c *False* d *True* e *False*
Gall bladder innervation remains intact with selective vagotomy. However, even after truncal vagotomy the evidence for increased incidence of gall-stones is not convincing.

*Complications of vagotomy*
These include:
1 *Post-operative dysphagia*. Usual onset of symptoms in second to third post-op week. Probably due to peri-oesophageal haematoma, with most resolving spontaneously, but some proceed to fibrous stricture.
2 *Gastric stasis*. Occurs after any type of vagotomy with inadequate drainage.
3 *Dumping syndromes*. Early dumping (10–20 minutes after a meal) due to rapid gastric emptying of hyperosmolar contents into jejunum and resultant sudden movement of extraluminal fluid into the gut.
  Late dumping (60–90 minutes after meal) due to reactive hypoglycaemia. Less common and less troublesome than early dumping.
4 *Post-vagotomy diarrhoea*. Most common with truncal vagotomy, less so with selective vagotomy and least common with HSV. Although some steatorrhoea occurs after vagotomy this is very rarely enough to cause nutritional consequences.
5 *Bilious vomiting*.
6 *Recurrent ulceration*. 5–10% after adequate vagotomy.
**REF: R17**

**A12**  a *True*  b *False*  c *True*  d *True*  e *True*

*Complications of partial gastrectomy*
These include:
1 *Gastro-oesophageal incompetence.* Causes reflux oesophagitis.
2 *Gastric incontinence.* The dumping syndromes — see **A11**.
3 *Duodenogastric reflux.* Causes bile vomiting and biliary gastritis. The long-term effects of gastritis include Intrinsic Factor deficiency and an increased prevalence of gastric cancer.
4 *Delayed gastric emptying.* Due to stomal stenosis (usually because of recurrent ulcer and resulting fibrosis) or torsion or herniation.
5 *Afferent loop syndrome* (Billroth 2). True syndrome rare — most ascribed symptoms are due to bile reflux. Obstructed afferent loop usually due to an internal herniation around the stoma.
6 *Recurrent ulcer.* Inadequate reduction of acid/pepsin secretion. Occasionally due to 'retained antrum' after Billroth 2 resulting in relative hypergastrinaemia.
7 *Anaemia.*
(a) Iron deficiency. Impaired absorption, or small blood losses from peristomal gastritis and oesophagitis.
(b) Vitamin B12 deficiency. Due to Intrinsic Factor deficiency as a consequence of long term biliary gastritis.
(c) Folate deficiency. Dietary in origin. Poor intake due to post-gastrectomy symptoms.
8 *Osteomalacia.* Mostly after Billroth 2. Due to malabsorption and poor dietary intake of Vitamin D. There is also an increase in *osteoporosis* following partial gastrectomy.
9 *Weight loss.* Usually due to poor dietary intake as a result of post-gastrectomy symptoms. Severe steatorrhoea is rarely due to the gastrectomy.
10 *Pulmonary tuberculosis.* The increase is possibly due to lack of inactivation of ingested organisms by gastric acid.
**REF: R18**


**A13**  a *False*  b *True*  c *True*  d *False*  e *False*
Congenital *hypertrophic pyloric stenosis* usually presents at 3–4 weeks of age. Male to female ratio is 4:1 and 50% are first born.
  Most patients have a palpable 'tumour'. In doubtful cases it has been practice to perform a barium meal. However, ultrasound has been shown to be useful, although there are

some false negatives. Thus barium meal may still be necessary.
REF: R19

A14    a *False*   b *True*   c *False*   d *False*   e *True*

Thickened small bowel folds may be localized or generalized and are predominantly due to submucosal oedema, thickening or infiltration.

1 *Oedema*. Hypoalbumenaemia, e.g. nephrotic syndrome, protein-losing enteropathy, chronic liver disease, acute ischaemia, radiotherapy, lymphangiectasia, (primary or secondary).
2 *Haemorrhage*. Traumatic or spontaneous (anticoagulants, clotting disorder, Henoch-Schonlein purpura).
3 *Inflammation*. e.g. Crohn's disease (early sign); infestation (e.g. giardia); tuberculosis; Whipple's disease.
4 *Neoplasm*. Carcinoid; lymphoma; mastocystosis; macroglobulinaemia.
5 *Others*. Eosinophilic gastroenteritis; amyloid. The small bowel folds are not typically thickened in uncomplicated coeliac disease unless there is severe hypoalbumenaemia.
REF: R14

A15    a *False*   b *True*   c *True*   d *False*   e *False*

Predominant or sole border of small intestine involved by the following lesions:

|  | Mesenteric | Antimesenteric |
| --- | --- | --- |
| Jejunal diverticulosis | + |  |
| Meckel's |  | + |
| Duplication cyst | + |  |
| Peritoneal metastases | + |  |
| Haematogenous metastases |  | + |
| Crohn's |  |  |
|   ulceration, sinuses | + |  |
|   pseudosacculation | +/− | + |
| Lymphoma | + |  |

REF: R20

# Gastrointestinal Tract and Adnexa 63

**A16**  a *True*  b *True*  c *False*  d *False*  e *False*

Small bowel strictures
These are associated with:
1 *Inflammation*.
  (a) Non-infective:
    Crohn's disease (**REF: R21**).
    Eosinophilic gastroenteritis. Idiopathic, but sometimes associated with atopic disease. Also recently described with scleroderma, polymyositis and dermatomyositis. Can affect stomach, small and large bowel. Peripheral eosinophilia and mucosal infiltration with eosinophils. Strictures; serosal disease with ascites.
    Non-granulomatous ulcerative jejuno-ileitis (see **A18**). May present with strictures.
  (b) Infective: tuberculosis, strongyloides.
2 *Ischaemia*. e.g. atheroma, vasculitis.
3 *Neoplasm*. Carcinoid (**REF: R22**), (marked mesenteric desmoplastic response); lymphoma; carcinoma; metastases.
4 *Iatrogenic*. Radiotherapy (**REF: R23**); enteric-coated potassium tablets.
5 *Extrinsic*. Mesenteric masses; adhesions.

**A17**  a *True*  b *False*  c *True*  d *False*  e *True*
Coeliac disease (also inflammatory bowel disease), is associated with splenic atrophy and functional hyposplenism. Renal oxalate calculi form when hyperoxaluria occurs secondary to oxalate overabsorption. The major site of oxalate absorption is the colon. Normally non-absorbable calcium salts are formed in the small intestine, but in steatorrhoea the intraluminal fatty acids 'mop up' the calcium and thus allow absorbable oxalates to enter the colon. Ileostomy precludes colonic oxalate absorption, but these patients have a lower urinary volume and pH and are at risk of uric acid and calcium stones (**REF: R24**).
  Giardiasis rarely causes radiological change. In heavy infestation there may be thickening of valvulae conniventes and non-specific changes of malabsorption. Unlike strongyloides infestation, strictures do not occur. Retroperitoneal fibrosis is commoner in Crohn's disease than ulcerative colitis, but is a complication of panproctocolectomy.

**A18**  a *True*  b *True*  c *True*  d *True*  e *False*
Bowel-related causes of *hypertrophic osteoarthropathy* include: coeliac disease; inflammatory bowel disease; cystic fibrosis;

64        Answers and Notes

chronic liver disease; GI malignancies. *Idiopathic chronic (nongranulomatous) ulcerative jejuno-ileitis* is a rare syndrome of heterogenous nature. All patients have intestinal ulceration and malabsorption, but may be divided into those with:
(a) proven coeliac disease who later relapse;
(b) villous atrophy unaffected by gluten withdrawal;
(c) a normal intervening mucosa;
(d) malignant histiocytosis of the bowel.
Most patients are in the second category. Apart from ulceration, strictures are a feature as a result of fibrous healing. The prognosis is very poor; two-thirds die within three years (**REF: R25**).

*Coeliac disease* is associated with an increased incidence of carcinoma and lymphoma of the small bowel, and carcinoma of the oesophagus. The associated lymphoma is malignant histiocytosis in 90%. Other associations include dermatitis herpetiformis — 60% of DH patients have villous atrophy.

A19    a *True*   b *False*   c *True*   d *True*   e *False*

**Polyposis syndromes**

Each histological type of solitary polyp has a multiple counterpart.

*Adenomas*
Familial adenomatous polyposis (FAP) — dominant. Carcinomas develop in early adult life. Adenomas do not develop until teens. Polyps also in stomach and duodenum (usually hamartomas in stomach).
    *Gardner's syndrome*: as for FAP plus osteomata of skull and facial bones, epidermoid cysts, soft tissue tumours of skin, desmoid tumours of abdominal wall and mesentery. May develop carcinoma of the peri-ampullary region of the duodenum.

*Hamartomas*
Peutz-Jegher's syndrome: polyposis (mostly small bowel, but also stomach and colon) plus mucocutaneous pigmentation. Usually presents with colicky abdominal pain or intermittent obstruction due to recurrent intussusception or, less commonly, chronic intestinal blood loss. The malignant potential is still debated, but there appears to be a slight increase in the

## Gastrointestinal Tract and Adnexa

incidence of colorectal, gastric and duodenal cancer as well as ovarian tumours.
*Juvenile polyposis*: familial or non-familial. Solitary polyps much commoner, and may be cured by auto-amputation.

*Hyperplastic/inflammatory*
Nodular lymphoid hyperplasia: seen in normal children, but associated with inflammatory bowel disease, immune deficiency or lymphoma in adults.
Polyps associated with ulcerative colitis: (a) Pseudopolyps during an acute severe attack. These are in fact mucosal islands. (b) With low-grade activity, inflammatory polyps (sessile, frond-like or occasionally pedunculated). (c) Post-inflammatory polyps in quiescent phase following an acute attack. These are small sessile or, characteristically, filiform.

*Canada-Cronkhite syndrome*
Polyps throughout GI tract caused by cystic change in mucosa. Associated with alopecia, nail and skin abnormalities.
**REF: R26, R14**

A20  **a** *False* **b** *True* **c** *False* **d** *True* **e** *False*
*Yersinia enterocolitica* is a Gram-negative rod. In children, infection causes acute enteritis with fever and diarrhoea. In adolescents and adults it causes acute terminal ileitis or mesenteric adenitis. This may mimic acute appendicitis or Crohn's disease.

Radiological features include:
1 Small bowel — spasm; nodularity of the terminal ileum due to hypertrophied lymphoid follicles; oedema; superficial ulceration of the terminal ileum.
2 Colon — superficial ulceration and spasm in the caecum adjacent to ileal disease; mild diffuse colitis resembling ulcerative colitis; aphthae.

Abscess and fistula formation, stenosis, and severe mural thickening do *not* occur.
**REF: R27**

A21  **a** *True* **b** *False* **c** *True* **d** *True* **e** *False*
Excluding neonates, the commonest cause of an 'acute

abdomen' in children less than 2 years old is intestinal obstruction, of which intussusception and strangulated hernia are the most important subgroups. (In children aged more than 2 years, acute appendicitis and undiagnosed pain/mesenteric adenitis are more frequent.) The peak incidence of intussusception is 6–12 months. Ileocolic region is the commonest site. Classical features are colicky abdominal pain, vomiting and blood-stained stools. The intussusception may be palpable. Contraindications (both relative and absolute) to attempted barium enema reduction include a history of symptoms longer than 24–36 hours, evidence of complete bowel obstruction, systemic toxicity, peritonism, young infants, and children over 2 years. In addition if, at barium enema, barium is seen to be tracking between intussusception and intussuscipiens ('dissection sign') (**REF: R28**), this is a sign of non-reducibility and an indication to discontinue attempts at reduction. A characteristic ultrasonographic appearance of intussusception has been described with concentric echogenic and echolucent rings (**REF: R29**). Henoch-Schonlein purpura occurs usually in 3–7 year olds and is associated with GI symptoms in 35–60% of cases (abdominal pain due to intramural haemorrhage, perforation, intussusception, obstruction). Although no apparent cause of intussusception is usually found in patients less than 2 years old, those over this age are more likely to have a Meckel's diverticulum, polyp, lymphoma or other, rarer, lesions at the apex. For this reason it is advisable to treat intussusception surgically in this age group.
**REF: R30**

**A22**   a *True*   b *True*   c *True*   d *True*   e *False*

*Proven and possible risk factors*
Low birth weight neonates; congenital heart disease; perinatal 'stress', i.e. anoxia, infection, respiratory distress; umbilical vessel catheterization (intestinal ischaemia).

*Pathogenesis*
Probably direct or indirect mucosal injury allows bacterial invasion and proliferation.

*Clinical manifestations*
Vomiting, distension, bloody diarrhoea. In more advanced cases there may be signs of peritonitis. Systemic signs of shock, which may or may not indicate perforation. Onset usually during the first five days of life.

## Gastrointestinal Tract and Adnexa

*Radiology*
Commonest early sign is dilatation of the small bowel, probably due to ileus (but note difficulty in distinguishing small and large bowel in neonate). May involve only a few loops which appear elongated. Loss of bowel wall definition. Pneumatosis intestinalis (linear or cystic. Linear gas is likely to be subserosal and is therefore evidence of more advanced disease). Most often affects ileum and colon, but may involve any part of gut including the stomach. Portal venous gas — may be transient; not necessarily an ominous sign.
'Persistent loop sign', i.e. persistence of a localized distended loop. Thought by some to mean imminent perforation and thus indicate surgery.

*Complications*
Pneumoperitoneum and septicaemia, shock and disseminated intravascular coagulation. Later — colonic strictures in up to 25% of survivors. Usually present at 2–12 weeks.
In Hirschsprung's disease a necrotizing enterocolitis may develop, usually in the aganglionic area, and is presumably related to obstruction.
**REF: R31**

**A23**   a *True*   b *True*   c *True*   d *False*   e *False*

*Systemic complications of ulcerative colitis*
1  *Nutritional and metabolic.* e.g. hypoalbumenaemia, anaemia, hypokalaemia. Amyloidosis (very rare).
2  *Arthritis and spondylitis.* See **A51** and **A52**. Also finger clubbing and hypertrophic osteoarthropathy.
3  *Liver and biliary abnormalities in inflammatory bowel disease* (IBD).
(a) Pericholangitis — essentially benign and probably the mild end of the spectrum of (b).
(b) Primary sclerosing cholangitis (PSC) (see **A30**).
(c) Bile duct carcinoma. With or without PSC. Not prevented by proctocolectomy. Very rare in Crohn's.
(d) Cholesterol gall-stones. Due to ileal dysfunction, i.e. ileal resection or extensive or long-standing ileal Crohn's. Incidence not increased in ulcerative colitis.
**REF: R32**
4  *Skin. Erythema nodosum* (also in Crohn's disease, *Yersinia enterocolitis* and malabsorption states); pyoderma

gangrenosum (occurs in very active ulcerative colitis); stomatitis; aphthous ulceration in the mouth.
5 *Eyes.* Uveitis and episcleritis.
6 *Blood vessels.* Venous thrombosis and thromboembolism; cutaneous vasculitis.
7 *Renal calculi.* 2–10% overall in IBD. Particularly common in ileostomy patients (urate stones). Oxalate stones in Crohn's with ileal resection or extensive ileal disease. See **A17**.
**REF: R33**

A24 a *True* b *False* c *True* d *False* e *True*
It is believed that pseudomembranous colitis is caused by an exotoxin of *Clostridium difficile*. Culture of the organism alone, though suggestive in the presence of typical colonic changes, is not absolutely diagnostic since there are non-toxigenic strains. Predispositions: broad-spectrum antibiotics, old age, debility, abdominal surgery, malignancy. The rectum is not usually spared.

*Plain film changes of pseudomembranous colitis:* Colonic 'thumbprinting'; haustral thickening; visible flat-topped plaques at the margin of the colon; small bowel dilatation; large bowel dilatation; toxic dilatation; intramural gas; ascites.

Barium enema is relatively contraindicated, there being evidence that the condition may be worsened, and perforation can occur.
**REF: R34**

A25 a *False* b *True* c *False* d *True* e *True*

'Cathartic colon' results from chronic abuse of irritant cathartics. Typical radiological features include:
  Loss of haustrations and bowel shortening, especially on the right side.
  Later the whole of the colon may be tubular, resembling chronic ulcerative colitis.
  Multiple inconstant areas of spasm (pseudostrictures)
  Rarely true strictures due to fibrosis.
  Superficial punctate mucosal ulceration.
  ✻'Backwash' ileitis.
  ✻ Differentiation radiologically and histologically from chronic 'burned-out' ulcerative colitis may be difficult.
  Pathologically — mucosal atrophy, degeneration of the

myenteric plexus, melancosis coli.
There is relative sparing of the rectum.
**REF: R35**

**A26** **a** *False* **b** *False* **c** *False* **d** *True* **e** *True*

*Acute colonic pseudo-obstruction (Ogilvie's syndrome)*
**1** *Idiopathic.*
**2** *Secondary to*: pneumonia; cardiac failure; renal failure; acute intra-abdominal infection; trauma; drugs (adrenergic blockers, anticholinergics, anti-Parkinsonian); metabolic (*low* serum potassium; low serum calcium).
*Radiology*:
(a) Gaseous dilatation of the colon — may be gross. Caecal perforation occurs in up to 15%.
(b) Fluid levels scant.
(c) Presence or absence of rectal gas is unhelpful.
(d) Preservation of haustral pattern.
(e) There may be transition from dilated to normal lumen at or distal to splenic flexure, with a gradual or sharp 'cut-off'. Sharp cut off mimics true obstruction — 'instant' contrast enema (water soluble or dilute barium) is indicated in suspected acute large bowel obstruction or pseudo-obstruction to prevent unnecessary laparotomy in the former and exclude an obstructing lesion in the latter (**REF: R36**).
**REF: R37**

*Chronic colonic pseudo-obstruction*
This occurs in a variety of conditions including: diabetes mellitus; myxoedema; progressive systemic sclerosis; dermatomyositis; dystrophia myotonica; multiple sclerosis; Parkinsonism; amyloidosis, etc. Idiopathic forms occur, sometimes associated with familial autonomic nervous system abnormalities.

**A27** **a** *False* **b** *True* **c** *False* **d** *True* **e** *False*
*Solitary rectal ulcer syndrome* is a benign condition most frequently affecting young adults. It usually presents with rectal bleeding, often with a change in bowel habit, and rectal pain.

Main radiographic features (Barium Enema): normal or; mucosal nodularity, polyp or polypoid thickening of a valve of Houston, rectal ulcer, stricture, granularity (like ulcerative colitis), i.e. non-specific.

## Answers and Notes

Defaecography may be useful to demonstrate internal rectal prolapse and the anorectal angle. The condition does not usually respond to corticosteroids.
REF: R38

A28   a *True*   b *True*   c *True*   d *False*   e *True*

The main features of the *irritable bowel syndrome* (IBS) are abdominal pain and change in bowel habit, but there is a wide clinical spectrum, e.g. some patients have pain as their predominant symptom; others have painless diarrhoea.

**1** *Abdominal pain:* 38–98% in various series in adults. Usually left lower quadrant or lower abdomen, but anywhere. Pain due to the irritable colon can mimic biliary pain. The pain follows food in up to 75%.

**2** *Bowel habit:* intermittent or continuous symptoms, diarrhoea, constipation (scybala, 'rabbit pellets'), or alternating diarrhoea/constipation.

**3** *Flatus:* upwards and/or downwards.

**4** *Weight:* usually steady or increasing, but 20% have lost more than 7 pounds in the last 6 months. Severe weight loss points to another diagnosis.

**5** *Nausea:* in 50%. But usually little or no vomiting.

**6** *Sigmoidoscopy:* often mucus. Spasm seen on insufflation with excessive pain which often mimics the patient's spontaneous pain. The same is true of barium enema examination.

Patients may exhibit changes in motility of small and large intestine.
REF: R39

A29   a *True*   b *False*   c *True*   d *True*   e *True*

*Gas in the biliary tract*

**1** *Emphysematous cholecystitis.* Approximately one-third of patients are diabetic. Usually restricted to gall bladder, but gas occasionally seen in bile ducts.

**2** *Passage of calculus.* Via a fistula or via the sphincter of Oddi. Triad of gall-stone ileus: — gas in the biliary tree + ectopic gall-stone + small bowel obstruction.

**3** *Surgery.* Choledocho- or cholecyst-enterostomy or sphincterotomy.

**4** *Endoscopic sphincterotomy.*

# Gastrointestinal Tract and Adnexa 71

5 *Malignancy*. Fistulation between biliary tract and duodenum or colon.
6 *Penetrating duodenal ulcer*.
7 *Physiological*. Lax sphincter in the elderly.
**REF: R40**

A30    **a** *False*   **b** *False*   **c** *True*   **d** *True*   **e** *True*
Primary sclerosing cholangitis (PSC) is of unknown aetiology and is characterized by an inflammatory fibrosis affecting the intra- and extra-hepatic biliary tree. There is a strong association with ulcerative colitis (especially total colitis) but there is no direct relationship of the outcome of PSC with the severity and clinical course of ulcerative colitis. There is a questionable weak association of PSC with Crohn's disease. PSC may progress to biliary cirrhosis. Adenocarcinoma of the bile ducts occurs with increased frequency in ulcerative colitis, with and without PSC. Other associations of PSC include Riedel's thyroiditis and retroperitoneal fibrosis.
**REF: R41**

A31    **a** *False*   **b** *False*   **c** *False*   **d** *False*   **e** *True*
The generally accepted upper limit of normal of the internal lumen of the common hepatic duct on ultrasound examination is 6 mm.
     Measurements on ultrasound and at direct cholangiography (ERC and PTC) do not correspond due to the following:
1 At ERC assessment is made following direct injection of contrast medium which distends the duct.
2 Measurements are often taken at the distal common bile duct at ERC (the widest part of the common duct) and at the proximal common duct at ultrasound examination.
3 Radiographic magnification.
4 Underestimation by ultrasound because of reverberation.
     A proximal extrahepatic duct that is normal prior to cholecystectomy will remain normal unless further pathology intervenes. Thus a common duct of calibre >6 mm warrants further investigation. The distal common bile duct does dilate after cholecystectomy.

Up to 30% of patients with choledocholithiasis have normal calibre extrahepatic (and intrahepatic) ducts. In common bile duct obstruction, increase in extrahepatic duct calibre precedes

dilatation of intrahepatic ducts and this is therefore a more sensitive test of obstruction. However, intrahepatic dilatation is more specific in indicating obstruction.
**REF: R42**

A32 **a** *True* **b** *True* **c** *True* **d** *False* **e** *False*
In simplistic terms bile consists of conjugated bile acids, cholesterol and phospholipids (lecithin), and conjugated bilirubin (pigment). The bile acids solubilize the cholesterol with the acid of lecithin. Gall-stones may occasionally consist purely of cholesterol or pigment, but the majority are of mixed constituents. About 10% contain enough calcium salts to be radio-opaque.

*Predisposing factors in the formation of gall-stones*
1 *Disturbance of the bile acid/cholesterol ratio* leading to saturation or supersaturation with cholesterol:
(a) Increased cholesterol concentration in bile: demographic; familial; dietary and hormonal factors. Obesity. Drugs (clofibrate, OCP).
(b) Diminished conjugated bile acids:
 (i) malabsorption of bile acids due to ileal disease (Crohn's disease); or ileal resection leading to a diminution of the bile acid pool.
 (ii) decreased synthesis of bile acids by the liver in chronic liver disease, e.g. alcoholic cirrhosis and primary biliary cirrhosis (PBC) (up to 40% prevalence of gall-stones in PBC).
2 *Pigment or mixed stones.*
(a) Chronic haemolysis.
(b) Stasis.
 (i) Congenital anomalies, e.g. choledochal cyst.
 (ii) Poor gall bladder function, e.g. diabetes mellitus, truncal vagotomy.
 (iii) Cystic fibrosis.
 (iv) Biliary infection.
In carcinoma of the gall bladder, about 80% of patients have co-existent gall-stones.
**REF: R43**

A33 **a** *True* **b** *False* **c** *True* **d** *False* **e** *False*
Ultrasound examination has at best a 50–60% sensitivity for common duct calculus visualization. Although ultrasound is

very good at detecting intra- and/or extra-hepatic bile duct dilatation, choledocholithiasis is the commonest cause of obstruction without dilatation (**REF: R42**). The serum biochemistry in cholestatic (i.e. intrahepatic cholestasis or extrahepatic obstructive) jaundice shows:
(a) predominantly conjugated hyperbilirubinaemia.
(b) urobilinogen is formed from conjugated bilirubin in the bowel and enters the enterohepatic circulation. Some is re-excreted through the liver; the rest in urine. If no bilirubin reaches the bowel, in bile duct obstruction, urobilinogen is absent from urine and faeces.
(c) elevated alkaline phosphatase.
(d) only minimal or mild increase in markers of hepatocellular damage such as transaminases.

Courvoisier's law states that if, in a patient with jaundice, the gall bladder is distended, the cause of jaundice is unlikely to be cholelithiasis.
**REF: R16**

A34    **a** *True*   **b** *True*   **c** *True*   **d** *False*   **e** *False*
Peri-ampullary duodenal diverticula are associated with an increased incidence of pancreaticobiliary disease and of recurrent choledocholithiasis following cholecystectomy (**REF: R44**). Complications of duodenal diverticula include the consequences of inflammation (sometimes associated with ectopic gastric mucosa), such as ulceration, perforation and haemorrhage. Abscess formation, duodenocolic fistulae and enterolith formation have also been reported.

In coeliac disease, low cholecystokinin levels are a cause of poor gall bladder emptying. Although ultrasound demonstration of dilatation of the portal vein (>12 mm) is fairly specific for portal hypertension, this sign is not very sensitive and, in a group of patients, the degree of dilatation does not correlate well with the severity of hypertension. However, a reduction of calibre has been demonstrated in individual patients in response to medical therapy. A more specific sign of portal hypertension is a lack of response of the portal vessels to respiration. Other ultrasound signs which may be present in portal hypertension — ascites, recanalization of the umbilical vein, varices, portal vein occlusion, splenic enlargement.
**REF: R45, R46**

A35    **a** *True*   **b** *True*   **c** *False*   **d** *False*   **e** *False*
Ultrasound is the initial investigation of choice in *Budd-Chiari*

syndrome (**REF: R47, R48**). Apart from ascites, more specific changes include the absence of the normal hepatic vein outflow into the inferior vena cava, and enlargement of the caudate lobe relative to the other liver lobes. In addition abnormal intrahepatic venous channels may be seen. Other imaging modalities of use are Tc-labelled colloid scintigraphy (marked increase in activity in the caudate lobe which is relatively non-specific); CT (ascites, enlarged caudate lobe, absence of opacification of hepatic veins with IV contrast, delayed and heterogeneous contrast uptake by the liver with prolonged enhancement of the periphery), and hepatic venography ('spider's-web' pattern) (**REF: R49**).

Various ultrasound patterns may be seen in *cavernous haemangioma*. In many cases the appearances are non-specific. Smaller lesions tend to be hyperechoic relative to normal liver and, as such, may be difficult to distinguish from some metastases. However, haemangiomas will often exhibit posterior acoustic enhancement, an appearance which is very specific. Contrast-enhanced CT in the cavernous haemangioma will demonstrate gradual 'filling-in' of the lesion with contrast medium on delayed scans taken up to several minutes after contrast injection. Delayed blood pool imaging with Tc-labelled erythrocytes is very sensitive and specific in the diagnosis of haemangiomas.
**REF: R50, R51, R52**

A36   a *False*   b *False*   c *False*   d *True*   e *True*

**Tc-IDA imaging**

The Technetium-labelled derivatives of iminodiacetic acid (IDA) are secreted into the bile after active transport across the hepatocytes.

Static images of the liver are obtainable in the initial phases of the study; note that the radionuclide is taken up by the hepatocytes (cf. the reticuloendothelial cells in colloid scintigraphy).

*Applications*
1  *Suspected acute cholecystitis* (**REF: R53**). Normally the common bile duct and intestinal activity is visible about 20 minutes after intravenous injection, and gall bladder visualization occurs at 20–40 minutes. Since the vast majority of cases of acute cholecystitis are associated with cystic duct obstruction, the gall bladder is not visualized in such cases. Normal visualization

within 60 minutes virtually excludes acute cholecystitis when the test is performed soon after the onset of symptoms. Non-visualization is very sensitive in the diagnosis but not totally specific since delayed demonstration may occur in some normals and in some patients with chronic cholecystitis. Therefore, delayed imaging should be performed up to 4 hours if the gall bladder is not seen within one hour (and up to 24 hours in selected cases with intercurrent diseases (**REF: R54**). Other causes of delayed or non-visualization include:
(a) prolonged fasting; parenteral nutrition;
(b) acute pancreatitis; alcoholism;
(c) severe intercurrent illness;
(d) hepatocellular dysfunction.
**2** *Testing biliary patency*. Although able to differentiate obstructive from non-obstructive jaundice with accuracy, the resolution of scintigraphy is not adequate for demonstration of cause and limits its use largely to (i) the post-surgical patient for testing the patency of *enterobiliary anastomoses* and (ii) neonatal jaundice, to help differentiate *neonatal hepatitis from biliary atresia* (**REF: R55**).
**3** *Detection of biliary leakage* following surgery, instrumentation or trauma (**REF: R56**).
**4** Delayed emptying in the *afferent loop syndrome*.
**5** *Assessment of duodenogastric reflux*.

*The ultrasound signs of acute cholecystitis*
These include:
**1** *Distended and spherical gall bladder*. Also seen in diabetes, post-surgery, prolonged biliary stasis, some causes of common bile duct (CBD) obstruction (Ca pancreas), narcotic administration, post vagotomy.
**2** *Thickened and oedematous wall*. 'Double wall sign' — anechoic layer sandwiched between echogenic layers. Other causes of gall bladder wall thickening include: chronic cholecystitis (usually a small gall bladder); ascites; acute hepatitis; cirrhosis; hypoalbumenaemia; congestive heart failure; adenomyomatosis and cholesterolosis.
**3** *Gall bladder calculi*. Occasionally an immobile stone is visualized in the neck of the gall bladder.
**4** *'Ultrasound Murphy's sign'*. Maximal tenderness when probe is applied over the gall bladder.

These signs mostly lack specificity, although in the appropriate clinical context Ultrasound is reliable in the confirmation of acute cholecystitis. Hepatobiliary radionuclide imaging is the gold-standard.

Complications of cholecystitis visible on Ultrasound: gangrenous cholecystitis; perforation and pericholecystic abscess; emphysematous

cholecystitis; empyema of gall bladder.
**REF: R57**

*Colloid scintigraphy in diffuse liver disease*
Abnormalities on colloid scintigraphy in most diffuse liver diseases include:
1 *Changes in liver size.* Usually enlargement, but shrunken liver occurs in long-standing cirrhosis.
2 *Irregular hepatic distribution of activity.*
3 *Diminished hepatic and increased extrahepatic colloid accumulation in spleen, bone marrow and lungs.* There is good correlation between the degree of liver dysfunction and accumulation of extrahepatic colloid.
4 *Sometimes hypertrophy of the left lobe of liver.* In severe alcoholic hepatitis there is typically virtually no uptake of radionuclide by the liver.

Besides fatty infiltration and cirrhosis, less common causes of diffuse liver disease, and hence the above changes, are: acute hepatic necrosis, congestive cardiac failure, biliary cirrhosis, leukaemia, diffuse lymphomatous infiltration, haemochromatosis, sarcoidosis, collagen diseases and bilharzia (**REF: R58, R59**).
In Budd-Chiari syndrome there is diffuse poor uptake of colloid, but with relative preservation centrally in caudate lobe. However, this may be seen in other diffuse liver diseases.

*Scintigraphy in gastrointestinal blood loss*
The site of intestinal blood loss can be determined by injecting intravenously Tc-labelled sulphur colloid, or Indium-labelled red cells, or by *in vivo* labelling of erythrocytes with methylene diphosphonate. It is claimed that rates of bleeding below 1 ml/minute can be detected. Meckel's diverticulum is an important source of intestinal blood loss in children. Heterotopic gastric mucosa is nearly always present under these circumstances (and in about one third of asymptomatic Meckel's), with resulting peptic ulceration. Sodium pertechnetate is taken up by eutopic and heterotopic gastric mucosa.
**REF: R59**

A37  a *False*  b *True*  c *True*  d *False*  e *True*
Haemochromatosis causes a generalized increase in density of the liver which may be recognizable on plain radiography, and is apparent on CT (which may be used to monitor progress on treatment).

## Gastrointestinal Tract and Adnexa 77

*Causes of intrahepatic calcification*
These include:
1 *Granulomatous and other infections*. TB; histoplasmosis; (rarely brucella, coccidiomycosis); healed pyogenic or amoebic abscess; Hydatid cyst (one to two thirds calcify within 5–10 years after infection. Calcified cysts may be active or inactive, but extensive calcification favours inactivity); Armillifer armillatus; chronic granulomatous disease of childhood.
2 *Neoplasms*. Hepatoma — calcification rare in adults, commoner in children. Haemangioma — spicular, radiating calcification. Metastases — colloid carcinomas of colon, osteosarcoma, ovary, thyroid, and many others rarely.
3 *Capsular calcification*. Previous pyogenic infection; meconium peritonitis; pseudomyxoma peritonei; trauma; alcoholic cirrhosis.
4 *Trauma*. Calcified haematoma.
5 *Vascular*. Thrombus in portal vein; aneurysm of hepatic artery.
6 *Biliary*. Gall-stones; porcelain gall bladder; limey bile.
**REF: R60**

A38   a *False*   b *False*   c *True*   d *False*   e *False*
The normal pancreas is of equal or greater echogenicity to normal liver at the same depth below the skin surface. Increasing echogenicity is seen with increasing age, probably due to atrophy of glandular tissue and replacement by echogenic fat and fibrous tissue. The main pancreatic duct is often seen with modern real-time ultrasound equipment. The normal calibre is usually taken to be 3 mm or less. Although ultrasound is widely used, CT is the imaging procedure of choice in severe acute pancreatitis, because overlying gas-containing stomach and loops of bowel obscure the region of the pancreas at ultrasound. Mild pancreatitis may be associated with an entirely normal ultrasound but typical findings are varying degrees of pancreatic enlargement and echolucency, which may be focal. Necrosis and fluid collection may be seen in severe disease. A major role of ultrasound is in the diagnosis and monitoring of pseudocyst, and, if indicated, in guiding diagnostic or therapeutic aspiration. Pseudocysts are very common after acute pancreatitis and up to 50% resolve spontaneously. Indications for aspiration are:
(a) The exclusion of pancreatic abscess/infected pseudocyst when there is clinical suspicion of sepsis.

(b) Progressive increase in size.
(c) Symptoms from mass effect of pseudocyst, e.g. obstructive jaundice.
**REF: R61, R62**

**A39**  a *True*  b *False*  c *True*  d *True*  e *False*

Up to two-thirds of cases of acute pancreatitis have normal plain films.

| Signs | Comments |
|---|---|
| Duodenal dilatation and/or fluid level | 42%, Useful sign |
| Gastric dilatation and fluid level | 29%, Useful sign |
| Small bowel dilatation, levels, 'sentinel loop' | Frequent but not specific |
| Colon dilated hepatic splenic flexure or transverse colon | Not specific and relatively infrequent |
| Pancreas | |
| calcification | Infrequent |
| separation of stomach & colon | Non specific (normal in obesity) |
| mottling in pancreatic bed | Rare but specific |
| Others e.g. absent left psoas left renal halo sign gasless abdomen | Relatively infrequent and not specific |

Chest radiograph abnormalities are frequent in severe acute pancreatitis (75%).
  Mainly left basal signs.
(a) Left pleural effusion in 43% in severe pancreatitis (5% in mild attacks).
(b) 'Shock lung' — ARDS — occasionally in severe pancreatitis.
**REF: R63**

**A40**  a *False*  b *True*  c *True*  d *False*  e *False*

*Causes of pancreatic calcification*
1  *Chronic pancreatitis due to alcohol*. Due to intraductal calculi. Very rare in pancreatitis due to biliary calculi.

2  *Cystic fibrosis.* A late feature.
3  *Following childhood malnutrition.* Result of kwashiorkor.
4  *Neoplasms.* Virtually never in adenocarcinoma, but about 10% of mucinous adenomas and adenocarcinomas. However, note that chronic calcific pancreatitis can co-exist with adenocarcinoma, there being an increased risk of carcinoma in chronic pancreatitis.
5  *Chronic pseudocyst.* May show curvilinear rim calcification.
6  *Hyperparathyroidism.* Note association between hyperparathyroidism, acute and chronic pancreatitis, hypercalciuria (nephrocalcinosis and renal calculi).
7  *Hereditary pancreatitis.*
**REF: R64**

A41  a *True*  b *True*  c *False*  d *False*  e *True*
Annular pancreas consists of a ring of pancreatic tissue completely or partly encircling the second part of the duodenum. Presentation may be at any age, or the condition may remain asymptomatic.

In the neonate the presentation is with duodenal obstruction within 24 hours of life. Diagnosis may be suggested by the 'double bubble' sign. Associated anomalies are duodenal stenosis or atresia, malrotation with peritoneal bands and intraduodenal diaphragm. There is an association with prematurity and (as with duodenal stenosis) Down's syndrome. Presentation in later childhood is rare. In the adult, symptoms are those of intermittent obstruction (vomiting and pain), or associated abnormalities. These associations include peptic ulcer, pancreatitis, and gall-stones. Sometimes presentation is from bleeding from the upper gastrointestinal tract. Obstructive jaundice also occurs, which may be related to gall-stones or pancreatitis exacerbating the pre-existing narrowing of the CBD due to the annular pancreas.
**REF: R16**

A42  a *True*  b *True*  c *False*  d *False*  e *False*

**Features of progressive systematic sclerosis (PSS)**

*Small bowel*
Hypomotility with varying degrees of dilatation and delayed transit. The valvulae conniventes are straightened and crowded

together ('hide bound' intestine). Sacculation with formation of pseudodiverticula occurs. Strictures are not seen.
Histologically, muscle is replaced by fibrous tissue. The villi are atrophic. Malabsorption is usually due to bacterial overgrowth, but vasculitis may be a contributing factor.

*Oesophagus*
Often part of the 'CREST' syndrome (Calcinosis, Raynaud's phenomenon, Esophageal involvement, Scleroderma, Telangiectasia). Diminished or absent peristalsis and dilatation. Incompetence of the lower oesophageal sphincter with reflux oesophagitis, peptic stricture, and sometimes Barrett's oesophagus. It is important to examine the patient in the recumbent position with a single swallow to detect aperistalsis, as the oesophagus can empty with the aid of gravity.

*Colon*
Slow transit, pseudosacculation, faecal impaction, episodes of pseudo-obstruction.

*Other features of PSS*
1  *Joints.* See **A47**.
2  *Lungs.* Basal interstitial fibrosis (with high incidence of adenocarcinoma of lung); chronic aspiration pneumonitis due to oesophageal involvement.
3  *Heart.* Cardiomyopathy; heart block and arrhythmias.
4  *Kidneys.* Renal failure due to nephrosclerosis.
**REF: R14**

**A43**  a *False*   b *False*   c *True*   d *True*   e *True*
Gastrografin is used in the treatment of meconium ileus because of its hyperosmolarity and meconium softening effects. The contrast medium is introduced rectally and refluxes under fluoroscopic control into the small bowel. In view of the hazards of hypertonic dehydration the following rules should be obeyed:
1  The patient should have uncomplicated meconium ileus (i.e. no volvulus, necrosis, perforation, peritonitis or atresia).
2  Fluid and electrolyte imbalance should be corrected prior to the procedure.
3  Intravenous infusion should be continued during and after the enema.
   With these criteria and good technique, up to 100% success rates have been reported.

Barium by mouth or via a small bowel tube is not contraindicated in small bowel obstruction, and may well clarify the site and cause (**REF: R65**). There is virtually no risk of converting a partial small bowel obstruction to a complete one, since barium remains fluid within the small intestine. However, suspected colonic obstruction is a contraindication to antegrade barium studies as barium may solidify and complete the obstruction. Barium enema is then the investigation of choice.

Contrast enema is absolutely contraindicated in acute dilatation (toxic dilatation) of the colon because of the risk of perforation. Plain abdominal radiography should be carried out in patients with acute colitis prior to a proposed barium enema, in order to exclude dilatation.

Because of its hyperosmolarity Gastrografin is contraindicated where there is a risk of aspiration into the lungs. Small quantities of barium, propyliodone (Dionosil), or non-ionic water-soluble contrast medium should be used.

Barium enema is relatively contraindicated after recent rectal or colonic biopsy via a rigid sigmoidoscope and should be delayed for 6–7 days (**REF: R66**). However, if the clinical indications are of sufficient urgency, the examination should be performed within this time interval with less distension than usual. Biopsies taken via a flexible instrument are superficial and barium enema may be performed immediately afterwards.

**A44**  a *True*  b *False*  c *False*  d *False*  e *True*
Pharmacological effects of glucagon include:
(a) Relaxation of the gastro-oesophageal sphincter. Oesophageal peristalsis is not affected, so that Buscopan is preferred in examination for varices.
(b) Reduction of gastric motility.
(c) Reduction of gastric acid and peptic secretion.
(d) Reduction of intestinal motility. However, there is intestinal hurry when the direct action of glucagon wears off, possibly due to an insulin rebound. Glucagon therefore acts as a small bowel hurrying agent.
(e) Effects on the biliary tract. Initial increase in tone of the sphincter of Oddi, followed by relaxation. Relaxation of the gall bladder. Increase in bile flow. Decrease in pancreatic secretion.

Glucagon should be avoided in patients with insulinoma (reactive hypoglycaemia) and in phaeochromocytoma (exacerbation of hypertension). Extremely rarely a patient has a history of hypersensitivity to glucagon.
**REF: R67**

**A45**  a *True*  b *True*  c *True*  d *False*  e *False*

*Causes of hypoalbuminaemia*
1 *Protein-losing enteropathy including*:
(a) Common. Ulcerative colitis; Crohn's disease.
(b) Occasional. Coeliac disease; carcinoma of stomach or colon; congestive heart failure; acute small bowel infections; dysentery.
(c) Rare. Lymphangiectasia; Ménétrièr's disease; Whipple's disease; tropical sprue; eosinophilic gastroenteritis; constrictive pericarditis; nodular lymphoid hyperplasia.
2 *Malabsorption.*
3 *Chronic liver disease.*
4 *Excess tubular loss*: nephrotic syndrome.

# Locomotor System

**A46** a *False*  b *False*  c *False*  d *True*  e *False*
*Gout* is characterized by assymetrical, eccentric soft tissue swelling, juxta-articular sharply defined erosions (tending to extend down the bone shaft), and relative lack of osteoporosis. The joint space remains intact early on in the disease. Gout does not produce erosions for at least 6 years from the onset of the symptoms. Calcification in soft tissue tophi is rare.
**REF: R68, R69, R70**

**A47** a *True*  b *True*  c *False*  d *False*  e *True*
*Sarcoid* of bone is associated with skin lesions and often involves the hand where signs include cyst formation which may affect the articular surface. Periarticular erosions are relatively common in primary and secondary *hyperparathyroidism*. About 20% with secondary disease have periarticular erosions in the hands. *Systemic sclerosis* is associated with a rheumatoid type arthritis in many patients (**REF: R71**). Polyarteritis nodosa and haemochromatosis are not associated with an erosive arthropathy. (See also notes to **A49**.)
**REF: R72**

**A48** a *True*  b *True*  c *True*  d *False*  e *False*
Systemic lupus erythematosus (SLE) is characterized by a non-erosive polyarthropathy of the hands with soft tissue changes including subluxations, ulnar deviation and hyperextension of the thumb. See notes to **A49** for Jaccoud's arthritis. Juvenile rheumatoid arthritis (RA) may cause ulnar deviation. Radial nerve injury will cause wrist-drop; median nerve injury may cause ulnar deviation with flexion against resistance.

Haemochromatosis is associated with chondrocalcinosis and a degenerative arthropathy with generalized joint space reduction, and a predeliction for 2nd and 3rd metatarsophalangeal joints. (See also notes to **A49** and **A50**.)
**REF: R70**

A49 a *False* b *True* c *False* d *True* e *True*

*Tuberose sclerosis* produces cystic changes in the phalangeal shafts, adjacent sclerosis and some periosteal reaction. Articular surfaces are not involved. *Sjogren's syndrome* consists of dry eyes, dry mouth and is usually part of rheumatoid disease. In *Jaccoud's arthritis* there are hand malalignments (especially ulnar deviation), due to peri-articular and fascial fibrosis following relapsing rheumatic fever. 'Hook erosions' are sometimes seen in relation to the metacarpal heads; these result from chronic ulnar deviation and are an adaptive response to stress (**REF: R73**). They are also seen in SLE, RA, old age and Parkinsonism. *Multicentric reticulohistiocytosis* is a 'lumpy bumpy' deposition arthritis — a destructive arthritis due to lipid containing macrophage deposition. Marginal erosions of the interphalangeal joints occur in up to 40% in *systemic sclerosis*. Erosions of the small joints (feet more than hands) occur in *Reiter's disease*; these start as marginal erosions or as diffuse loss of cortical definition in and adjacent to the joints. Occasionally progression to a destructive arthritis is seen. Periosteal reaction is a feature (**REF: R74**).

**Erosive arthritis involving multiple joints**
*Inflammatory*

| Rheumatoid arthritis | Rheumatoid type +/− Rh factor | Seronegative arthritides | Metabolic deposition |
|---|---|---|---|
| RA | Scleroderma | Ankylosing spondylitis | 'Lumpy-bumpy': |
|  | SLE | Reiter's | Gout |
|  | Psoriasis |  | Amyloidosis |
|  |  | Inflammatory bowel disease | Hyperlipidaemia |
|  |  | Juvenile chronic arthritis | Multicentric reticulohistio-cytosis |

*Degenerative*
'*Erosive osteoarthrosis*'. A contentious entity; a small number of primary osteoarthrosis patients have degenerative cysts which erode into the articular surface of the small joints of the hand and give a radiological picture of an erosive arthritis.

## Locomotor System

*Others*
Including sarcoid, hyperparathyroidism, haemophiliac joints.
**REF: R70, R75, R76, R71**

A50   **a** *False*   **b** *True*   **c** *False*   **d** *True*   **e** *True*

Distinguishing features of RA and seronegative polyarthritides*

|  | RA | Seronegative |
|---|---|---|
| *Joint involvement* | | |
| Symmetrical | usual | – |
| Assymetrical/random | – | typical |
| Only large joints | – | + |
| Bony ankylosis | – | + |
| *Spine* | | |
| Sacro-iliac joints | – | very strong HLA-B27 association |
| Lumbar spine with ankylosis | – | ditto |
| *Soft tissues* | | |
| Periarticular swelling | typical | |
| Diffuse swelling | | typical |
| Enthesopathy† | | typical |
| e.g. Calcaneal spurs | | |
| *Bone density* | | |
| Periarticular porosis | typical | +/– |
| *Periosteal reaction* | rare | + |
| *Serum factors* | | |
| HLA-B27 | – | strong |
| Rh. factor | + | – |
| Antinuclear Ab. | sometimes | – |

**REF: R70, R77**
* The American literature, in particular, uses the term 'rheumatoid variant' to denote the seronegative (spondylo) arthritides — psoriatic, ankylosing spondylitis, Reiter's, and that associated with inflammatory bowel disease.
† Enthesopathy is an abnormality of the sites of ligament and tendon attachments to bone
**REF: R78**

A51   **a** *True*   **b** *False*   **c** *False*   **d** *False*   **e** *True*
A high prevalence of HLA-B27 positivity is seen in:

(a) the spondyloarthritides, i.e. ankylosing spondylitis (>90%), Reiter's syndrome, psoriatic arthritis, colitis-associated spondyloarthritis. There is no association of HLA-B27 and inflammatory bowel disease as a group, but this association is strong when spondyloarthritis is present.
(b) patients developing reactive arthritis to yersinia, salmonella and gonococcus among other infections.
(c) some patients with juvenile chronic arthritis — those with a spondylitis type of clinical picture.
**REF: R79, R80**

**A52**    a *False*    b *False*    c *True*    d *True*    e *True*
Spondyloarthritis accompanies ulcerative colitis and Crohn's disease in about 10%. The changes in the spine are similar to classical ankylosing spondylitis rather than those found in the other spondyloarthritides. (Psoriatic spondylitis is typically associated with large, assymetrical syndesmophytes, paravertebral ossification; vertebral body squaring and involvement of apophyseal joints is unusual.)

The severity of the peripheral arthritis parallels the bowel disease activity whereas the spondylitis appears to be independent of it. The peripheral joints most often affected are medium sized joints, especially knees. Radiographs of peripheral joints usually show effusion and soft tissue swelling only.

Infective enterocolitis or dysentery may be accompanied by arthritis in one or more joints. Peripheral arthritis takes three forms: (a) 'reactive' with an effusion visible only; (b) progression to Reiter's syndrome; (c) rarely, septic arthritis.
**REF: R81, R82**

**A53**    a *False*    b *False*    c *False*    d *True*    e *True*
Ankylosing spondylitis is commoner in males. Age of onset 15–30 years. Associations: iritis; aortic regurgitation (but rarely mitral); cardiac conduction defects; amyloidosis; atlanto-axial subluxation or spinal fractures; apical pulmonary fibrosis with cyst formation; cauda equina syndrome.
**REF: R83**

**A54**    a *True*    b *False*    c *False*    d *False*    e *True*
Causes of bilateral sacroiliitis:
(a) The spondyloarthritides: ankylosing spondylitis; Reiter's;

Locomotor System 87

psoriasis; ulcerative colitis and Crohn's disease.
(b) Intestinal lipodystrophy (Whipple's disease).
(c) Behcet's (see **A86**).
(d) Juvenile chronic arthritis — HLA-B27 associated.
(e) PVC workers (also acro-osteolysis).
(f) Gout (**REF: R84**).
Forestier's disease is distinguished from ankylosing spondylitis, by the continuous periosteal reaction ('candle guttering') seen mainly on the anterior surface of the dorsal spine and the absence of sacro-iliitis, and the different clinical picture. It is painless, occurs in the middle-aged and elderly and has an association with diabetes.
**REF: R70**

A55 a *True* b *False* c *True* d *True* e *False*
The crystal deposition diseases include:
(a) Gout (monosodium urate).
(b) Pseudogout (calcium pyrophosphate).
(c) Hydroxyapatite deposition disease (HADD).
HADD may be primary (idiopathic) or secondary to collagen vascular disease (especially scleroderma), renal failure/secondary hyperparathyroidism, or osteoarthrosis. Deposition is usually *periarticular* (but may be intra-articular) causing peri-arthritis, calcific tendonitis or bursitis. Symptoms in the three crystal-associated diseases may be similar. Anything from acute synovitis to joint destruction can be seen in HADD, but it may be asymptomatic.
**REF: R85, R86**

A56 a *True* b *False* c *False* d *False* e *False*
*Chondrocalcinosis* (calcification within hyaline or fibro-cartilage) has been described in association with: hyperparathyroidism; gout; pseudogout; haemochromatosis; ochronosis; degenerative arthritis; Wilson's disease; acromegaly; hypophosphatasia; diabetes mellitus, and other conditions.
Radiological changes of *Wilson's disease* include diffuse demineralization, premature osteoarthrosis with subchondral bone fragmentation and sclerosis. Articular calcifications are seen. Multiple ossicles, especially around the wrist, simulate those seen in Vitamin D-resistant rickets.
**REF: R86, R87**

**A57** **a** *True* **b** *True* **c** *True* **d** *False* **e** *False*

Widening of the intercondylar notch is part of the 'hyperaemic joint syndrome'. This mechanism is common to haemophilia, juvenile polyarthropathy and tuberculous arthritis. The radiological changes in the joints in *haemophilia* depend on the number of bleeding incidents. Progression occurs from osteoporosis and increased size of epiphyses due to hyperaemia, to joint space narrowing, subchondral cysts, marginal erosions and, later, secondary degenerative changes. Growth disturbances are probably related to hyperaemia and include premature epiphyseal fusion, abnormal modelling, squaring of the patella and broadening of the intercondylar notch.

*Juvenile polyarthritis* may produce a similar appearance. *Tuberculous arthritis* leads to the 'Phemister triad' of juxta-articular osteoporosis, marginal osseous erosions and gradual joint space narrowing. The differential diagnosis of the X-ray finding of an 'erosive arthropathy' involving a single joint with a relatively intact joint space suggests: tuberculous arthritis; gout; pigmented villonodular synovitis.
**REF: R75**

**A58** **a** *True* **b** *True* **c** *False* **d** *False* **e** *True*

The list of causes of *avascular necrosis* is vast. They may broadly be divided as follows (this is not a comprehensive list):
1 *Causes within the lumen of the blood vessels.* e.g. Thromboembolic disease; sickle cell disease; corticosteroid therapy; caisson disease; acute and chronic relapsing pancreatitis (due to fat embolism).
2 *Disease of the vessel wall.* e.g. Vasculitides such as polyarteritis nodosa, systemic lupus erythematosus, rheumatoid arthritis, sarcoidosis; arteriosclerosis.
3 *Disease of bone adjacent to vessels.* e.g. Infiltrations such as Histiocytosis X; Gaucher's disease; osteomyelitis; metastases.
4 *Traumatic.* Following subcapital fractures and dislocations; slipped femoral epiphysis.
5 *Idiopathic.* Osteochondroses — Perthes' disease.
**REF: R88, R89**

**A59** a *False* b *True* c *False* d *False* e *False*

|  | Perthes' | Slipped femoral epiphysis |
|---|---|---|
| Sex | M >F | M slightly > F |
| Age | 3–14 | 9–17 |
|  | Peak 6–8 | Peak 12 (F), 13 (M) |
| Bilateral | 15% (not concurrent) | 20–30% |

There is a tendency to retarded skeletal maturation in children with Perthes' disease, especially in boys. Recovery is usually more complete in younger children who develop the disease.
**REF: R88**

**A60** a *False* b *True* c *True* d *True* e *False*
The earliest signs of infections of the spine are reduction in disc space with areas of rarefaction of the end plates of the two adjacent vertebrae.

In *pyogenic* spondylitis, new bone/sclerosis with little destruction, is a feature. In *tuberculous spondylitis* the radiological appearances often differ in white and non-white patients:

| White | Non-white |
|---|---|
| No new bone/sclerosis Paravertebral abscess more common than in pyogenic infection | Often new bone/sclerosis Unusual variants (see below) |

Unusual variants of tuberculous spondylitis in non-whites include:
(a) Subligamentous spread below the anterior spinal ligament forming 'gouge defects' like those seen in lymphoma and aortic aneurysm, with relative sparing of the disc spaces.
(b) Primary involvement of pedicles.
(c) Collapse of a single vertebral body with sparing of the disc

space resembling secondary malignancy.
**REF: R90, R91, R92**

**A61**   **a** *False*   **b** *False*   **c** *False*   **d** *False*   **e** *True*

*Chordoma*
1. Chordoma is a neoplasm that arises from remnants of the primitive notochord.
2. Age distribution 30–70 years but mostly >50.
3. Site — Sacro-coccygeal 50%
   — Base of skull (clivus) 30%
   — Elsewhere in spine about 20% but especially C2
4. Locally malignant — metastases in < 10%
5. Radiologically appear as destructive or expanding lesions.
6. Calcification occurs in about half. A soft tissue mass (with or without calcification) is common. Chordoma may cross the intervertebral disc space.
7. Histology shows cords of regular clear cells with typical intracytoplasmic vacuoles.

**REF: R93, R94**

**A62**   **a** *True*   **b** *True*   **c** *False*   **d** *False*   **e** *True*

Site of some benign tumours and tumour-like lesions in the spine

| Vertebral body | Appendages |
|---|---|
| | Benign osteoblastoma (usually) |
| | Osteoid osteoma |
| | Chondroma |
| Haemangioma ──────────▶ | May extend |
| May extend ◀────────── | Aneurysmal bone cyst |
| Eosinophilic granuloma (histiocytosis X) | |
| Giant cell tumour | |

Giant cell tumours rarely occur in the spine, but when present are most often sacral. 20% of aneurysmal bone cysts and up to 50% of benign osteoblastoma occur in the spine. Aneurysmal bone cysts are unusual in their ability to cross the intervening disc and involve adjacent vertebrae.

Locomotor System 91

When *vertebra plana* occurs under the age of 15 years the commonest cause is Histiocytosis X. The incidence is greatest in the lumbar spine. The disc space is preserved, providing a valuable discriminator from infection, although there may be some paravertebral soft tissue swelling. Differential diagnosis of vertebra plana includes trauma, Gaucher's disease, lymphoma, leukaemia, osteoporosis, neurofibromatosis and Ewing's tumour.
REF: R95, R96, R97

A63   a *False*   b *True*   c *True*   d *True*   e *False*

*Causes of posterior scalloping of vertebral bodies*
Achondroplasia; mucopolysaccharidoses; neuro-fibromatosis (dural ectasia or neurofibroma — see A68); Marfan's syndrome; Ehlers-Danlos syndrome; acromegaly; severe and/or chronic communicating hydrocephalus; syringomyelia; tumours of spinal canal (but note uncommon with meningioma); idiopathic, etc.

*Spinal changes in mucopolysaccharidoses*
Hurler's syndrome — posterior scalloping, ovoid vertebral bodies, with anterior inferior beak. Hypoplastic upper lumbar body/bodies.
  Morquio's syndrome — generalized vertebra plana, hypoplastic dens, hypoplastic upper lumbar vertebral bodies. Central beaking of vertebral bodies (mnemonic — 'm' for middle beak and Morquio).
REF: R88

A64   a *True*   b *True*   c *False*   d *False*   e *False*
The following are causes of *atlanto-axial subluxation:*
1 Trauma.
2 Inflammatory. Atlanto-axial subluxation, in association with the arthritides, is usually due to pannus derived from synovial bursae adjacent to the odontoid peg. This weakens the strap-like transverse ligament which runs behind the peg. The distance between the anterior arch of the atlas and the odontoid peg should not exceed 3 mm in adults. Radiographs in flexion may be needed to demonstrate widening in some cases. In children the distance may normally be greater than in adults. Rheumatoid disease and ankylosing spondylitis are the commonest causes in adults. Other inflammatory causes

include systemic lupus erythematosus and psoriatic arthritis.
In children, seropositive chronic arthritis and retropharyngeal abscess (causing soft tissue laxity) cause subluxation.
**3** *Congenital syndromes.* Congenital absence of anterior arch of atlas or odontoid. Down's syndrome. Morquio's disease.
**REF: R88**

**A65**    **a** *True*   **b** *True*   **c** *True*   **d** *False*   **e** *True*
Most patients present with pain especially associated with fractures. Those with facial bone lesions tend to have swelling +/− pain.
Lesions in long bones tend to be diaphyseal or diametaphyseal. Polyostotic disease is associated with café-au-lait pigmentation and various endocrine disorders, notably sexual precocity (in females, Albright disease) and thyroid disease. Sex incidence is approximately equal overall, but Albright's is very rare in males.
Malignant change is rare and is usually due to fibrosarcoma. Lesions which have been present for many years may exhibit dense calcification within.
Polyostotic fibrous dysplasia is typically predominantly unilateral in the limbs.
**REF: R98, R99**

**A66**    **a** *True*   **b** *False*   **c** *False*   **d** *True*   **e** *True*
*Marfan's syndrome* and *homocystinuria* resemble each other. Both are inherited disorders of collagen. Comparison of features:

|  | Marfan's | Homocystinuria |
|---|---|---|
| Arachnodactyly | + | + |
| Scoliosis | + | + |
| Osteoporosis | − | + |
| Lens dislocation | +↑ | +↓ |
| Mental retardation | − | common |
| Aortic incompetence | + | − |
| dilatation/dissection | + | − |
| Mitral valve prolapse | + | − |
| Thrombosis artery & vein | − | + |
| Avascular necrosis of bone | − | + |
| Joint mobility | increased | decreased |
| Enlarged vertebrae & femoral heads | − | + |

**REF: R100, R101**

Locomotor System 93

**A67**   a *False*   b *False*   c *False*   d *True*   e *True*

The radiographic changes in *thalassaemia* are due to marrow hyperplasia and extramedullary haemopoiesis. Marrow hyperplasia, both in normal sites of haemopoiesis and others not normally the site of such activity, e.g. phalanges, results in widening of the medullary cavity, cortical thinning, and widening of the intertrabecular spaces (causing a coarsened pattern). Secondary changes include enlargement of vascular channels, abnormal bone modelling and premature epiphyseal fusion.

The skull shows widening of the diploic space and the classical 'hair-on-end' appearance.* There is sparing of the occiput and base of skull due to the lack of marrow in these areas.

The facial bones undergo marrow hyperplasia with resultant lack of pneumatization of the sinuses and, sometimes, hypertelorism. Extramedullary soft tissue haemopoiesis is seen as paravertebral soft tissue swellings, and subperiosteal deposits. Patients with pure thalassaemia, unlike those with sickle cell disease, are not prone to bone ischaemia and salmonella osteomyelitis.

\* Other causes of 'hair-on-end' appearance in the skull:
   Congenital haemolytic anaemias
   Iron deficiency anaemia in childhood
   Cyanotic congenital heart disease
   Childhood polycythaemia vera
   NB, Neuroblastoma metastases cause spiculated periosteal reaction in addition to other signs — sutural widening and osteolytic areas.

**REF: R102**

**A68**   a *True*   b *True*   c *False*   d *False*   e *True*

The skeletal manifestations of *neurofibromatosis* are mainly due to mesodermal dysplasia.

1   *Skull*. Defect in the postero-superior wall of the orbit — 'bare orbit'. Optic canal enlargement — optic nerve glioma. Occipital defects.

2   *Spine*. Dural ectasia producing posterior scalloping of vertebral bodies and pedicle erosions. Intervertebral foraminal enlargement due to neurofibroma. Posterior paraspinal mass — usually due to lateral meningocele rather than neurofibroma. Kyphoscoliosis — usually short segment and progressive.

3   *Ribs*. Twisted ribbon deformity. Notching — due to neurofibromas.

94  Answers and Notes

4 *Extremities*. Streaky bone texture. Increase in length and subperiosteal haematoma (cirsoid neurofibroma). Overtubulation (plexiform neurofibroma). Bowing and pseudoarthrosis. Marginal cortical defects. Intramedullary lesions — neurofibromas, non-ossifying fibromas, etc.

Neurofibromatosis is a cause of hypophosphataemic osteomalacia (see **A83**).
**REF: R103, R104**

**A69**  a *False*  b *True*  c *False*  d *True*  e *False*
Congenital syndromes with a small acetabular angle include:
*Achondroplasia* (small pelvis, short ilia, narrow sacrum, slit-like greater sciatic notch, low sacro-iliac joints, squared iliac wings and flat acetabular angles). 'Champagne glass pelvis' (normal is brandy glass shape).

*Down's syndrome* (flared iliac wings, flat acetabula, hypoplastic ischia, reduced iliac index = half the sum of both iliac and acetubular angles — valid only in first year).

Also prune-belly syndrome; osteogenesis imperfecta; arthrogryposis; exstrophy of the bladder.

In *Morquio's syndrome* (and to a lesser extent in Hunter's and Hurler's (mucopoly-saccharidoses) the pelvis exhibits an increase in acetabular angle, rounded iliac crests and low articulation of sacrum ('wine glass pelvis'). Specific pelvic abnormalities are not seen in *Turner's syndrome* — an android pelvic inlet may be present, and there is delayed skeletal maturation. In *congenital hypothyroidism* (cretinism) there is delayed appearance and fusion of epiphyses; the hips show delayed and stippled ossification of the femoral capital epiphysis followed by fragmentation and secondary changes in the acetabulum.

**A70**  a *False*  b *True*  c *False*  d *True*  e *False*

*Fusion of carpal bones*
**1** *Congenital*.
(a) Isolated abnormality. Usually only two bones and in same carpal row. Triquetral-lunate is the commonest. May be familial. Much more common in Blacks. F:M ratio 2:1.
(b) Part of a more generalized skeletal disorder. Often involves multiple bones and extends across rows, e.g. Ellis-van Crefeld syndrome (chondroectodermal dysplasia); dyschondrosteosis

Locomotor System 95

(with Madelung's deformity); symphalangism; diastrophic dwarfism; acrocephalosyndactyly (Apert's syndrome — includes craniostenosis); arthrogryposis.
(c) Part of a primarily non-skeletal disorder. Turner's syndrome; Holt-Oram syndrome; Hand-foot-uterus.
**2** *Acquired.* Post-surgical. Inflammatory disease — especially post-infective (tuberculous), juvenile chronic arthritis, psoriasis, rheumatoid arthritis
**REF: R105, R106**

A71  **a** *True*  **b** *True*  **c** *False*  **d** *False*  **e** *True*
In *achondroplasia* the spinal canal demonstrates progressive narrowing of the interpedicular distances and also narrowing in the anteroposterior plane. The vertebral bodies are flattened and there is an increase in height of the disc spaces. The association of colonic polyposis and osteomas constitutes *Gardner's syndrome* (see **A19**).

*Multiple naevoid basal cell carcinomas*, odontogenic keratocysts of the mandible and maxilla and other findings (most commonly rib and vertebral anomalies, mental retardation, ocular lesions and lamellar calcification of the falx) are seen in basal cell naevus syndrome (Gorlin's syndrome) (**REF: R106**).

A72  **a** *False*  **b** *False*  **c** *True*  **d** *False*  **e** *True*
*Secondary deposits expanding bone:*
  Thyroid carcinoma
  Renal adenocarcinoma
  Phaeochromocytoma
  Malignant melanoma
  Myeloma
  Rarely bronchial and breast carcinoma in flat bones.
**REF: R88, R107, R108, R109**

A73  **a** *True*  **b** *False*  **c** *True*  **d** *True*  **e** *True*
*Primary malignancies producing osteoblastic deposits in bone*
  Prostate
  Breast — usually after treatment, occasionally before
  Lymphoma
  Mucoid adenocarcinoma, e.g. stomach, colon
  Carcinoid tumour
  Bronchus occasionally

Bladder occasionally
Leukaemia especially after anti-folate metabolite treatment
Medulloblastoma
Multiple myeloma rarely (see **A78**).
Many other carcinomas can rarely give osteoblastic metastases, e.g. pancreas, larynx.
**REF: R88**

**A74**    **a** *False*   **b** *False*   **c** *True*   **d** *True*   **e** *False*
*Chondromyxoid fibroma* rarely exhibits matrix calcification, unlike other benign cartilage tumours. There is often endosteal sclerosis and scalloping. They tend to lie eccentrically in the metaphysis. Epiphyseal involvement is very uncommon. *Benign osteoblastomas* exhibit matrix mineralization in up to 50%. *Chondroblastomas* are epiphyseal in origin (and may extend to, and erode, the subarticular cortex) but often extend into the metaphysis. Matrix calcification is common. They are well-defined with a thin sclerotic rim. Periosteal reaction adjacent to the lesion may be seen (see also table following **A76**).
**REF: R110, R111, R112**

**A75**    **a** *False*   **b** *False*   **c** *False*   **d** *True*   **e** *True*
Osteoid osteoma is fairly common in the spine occurring usually in the neural arch. The classical appearance is of a small radiolucent nidus (the actual osteoid tumour) which may contain a diagnostic central calcified portion. Sclerotic bone surrounds the nidus. However, in cancellous bone and in sub-periosteal locations, the sclerosis is often absent.
    Diagnosis may be elusive. Tomography may be required for visualization. Bone scintigraphy is useful where radiography is negative in the presence of a suggestive history. These lesions are 'hot'. Angiography is sometimes required to demonstrate a nidus.
    The pain of osteoid osteoma is classically nocturnal and relieved by aspirin (see also table following **A76**).
**REF: R113**

**A76**    **a** *True*   **b** *False*   **c** *True*   **d** *True*   **e** *False*
50% of *enchondromas* occur in the hands. It is extremely rare for lesions in the hands to undergo malignant change. Axial lesions have much higher malignant potential. Patients with multiple

Locomotor System 97

lesions have a higher statistical risk of malignancy.
*Chondrosarcomas* may arise *de novo* or secondary to enchondromas or exostoses. Primary lesions are more common. Maffucci's syndrome consists of multiple enchondromas, with resultant dwarfism and deformity of the affected limb, and associated (cavernous) haemangiomatosis (containing phleboliths). Sarcomatous change may develop. *Dyschondroplasia* (Ollier's disease) is characterized by persisting cartilage masses in metaphyses and diaphyses, subperiosteal deposition of cartilage, and exclusive or predominant unilateral involvement. The affected bones often show deformity and shortening. Rarely chondrosarcomatous degeneration may occur.

Sarcomatous change in *diaphyseal aclasis* occurs in up to 20%, and is nearly always to chondrosarcoma.

**REF: R114**

Age distribution and site of commoner benign bone lesions

| Lesion | Peak age | Commonest bones | Site within bone* |
|---|---|---|---|
| Enchondroma | 10–50 | hands, feet 60% long bones 20% flat bones 20% SINGLE OR MULTIPLE | M |
| Osteochondroma | 10–20 | tubular bones SINGLE OR MULTIPLE | M |
| Chondroblastoma | 10–20 | long bones | E |
| Chondromyxoid fibroma | 10–30 | lower limb tibia 50% | M |
| Osteoid osteoma | 10–20 | femur, tibia, spine | proximal D appendages |
| Osteoblastoma | 7–20 | spine 30–50% long bones | appendages M or D |
| Non ossifying fibroma | 8–20 | around knee | M |
| Monostotic fibrous dysplasia | 0–20 | femur, tibia flat bones | D or D/M |
| Giant cell tumour | 20–40 | long bones | subarticular |
| Haemangioma | increasing with age | spine, skull SINGLE OR MULTIPLE | Vertebral body |
| Aneursymal bone cyst | 10–30 | limbs, sacrum, spine | M, appendages |
| Simple bone cyst | 5–15 | proximal humerus/femur | M at first |
| Brown tumour | 40–60 | mandible, pelvis, ribs | various |
| Eosinophilic granuloma | <10 | skull, flat bones spine, long bones | D |
| Fibrous cortical defect | 4–8 | distal femur | M |

*E = epiphysis; M = metaphysis; D = diaphysis.

REF: R88, R96, R98, R110–113, R115, R116

A77    a *True*   b *False*   c *False*   d *True*   e *False*

Direct extension of a metaphyseal lesion across epiphyseal cartilage is unusual. When this is present it suggests infection or aggressive tumour. Some cartilage tumours cross the physis, notably chondroblastoma (of epiphyseal origin) and, occasionally, chondromyxoid fibroma. However, enchondromas do not involve the epiphysis prior to closure of the growth plate. Although primary aneurysmal bone cysts were thought to only very rarely cross into the epiphysis, a recent study has suggested otherwise (**REF: R117**).

Tuberculous osteomyelitis, by the time of presentation, may have crossed the physis. Patients present earlier with pyogenic bone infection, and, in all but young infants, the growth plate acts as a temporary barrier to spread from the usual focus in the metaphysis.

Extension of osteosarcoma across an open epiphyseal plate has been reported to occur in 75%. Giant cell tumour is subarticular in site in adults. It occurs very rarely prior to growth plate closure, and then abutts the plate.

A78    a *True*   b *False*   c *False*   d *False*   e *False*

*The radiological patterns of multiple myeloma*
These often occur in combinations.
1   Diffuse osteopenia.
2   Accentuation of trabecular pattern in the axial skeleton (similar to other diseases where there is proliferation of marrow elements). The vertebral pedicles tend to be spared in myeloma (cf. metastases).
3   Punched out lesions — may produce endosteal scalloping, especially in the skull and long bones.
4   Diffuse bone destruction.
5   Expanding lesions, especially flat bones.
6   Bone sclerosis — occurs in 3%. In 37% of these the osteosclerosis is diffuse. This rare variant is associated with peripheral neuropathy. Sclerosis also follows chemotherapy.
7   Soft tissue masses, especially paraspinal and extrapleural.
8   The bones may appear radiographically normal. There is a suggestion that this is associated with poor prognosis — not

# Locomotor System

enough time for abnormalities to develop in a rapidly progressive disease.
9  Changes of amyloidosis, e.g. joint involvement.

Hypercalcaemia occurs in about 40%. Spinal cord compression may occur without vertebral collapse, presumably related to soft tissue masses. Radiography is more sensitive than bone scintigraphy in demonstrating the lesions of myeloma on a site-by-site basis. Scintigraphy is particularly insensitive in the skull. It performs better than radiography in only a few sites, e.g. ribs. 'Hot' lesions on radionuclide studies are associated with more active disease than 'cold'.
**REF: R118–R121**

A79  a *True*  b *False*  c *False*  d *False*  e *False*

*Radiological appearances of giant cell tumour*
This occurs after epiphyseal closure (very rarely before). Most are around the knee. They are typically subarticular and, especially in the early stages, eccentrically placed. There is an expanding zone of translucency. Gradual transition zone between normal and abnormal bone. Little or no periosteal reaction.
   Appearances are modified by surgery, fracture or radiotherapy. Some become malignant or are malignant from the outset. Accurate prediction of behaviour from histology is difficult. Tumours may be locally malignant and/or give rise to lung metastases. Local extension into soft tissues is not necessarily a sinister feature.
**REF: R116**

A80  a *False*  b *True*  c *True*  d *True*  e *False*
Most patients with typical *intramedullary osteosarcoma* are between 10 and 25 years old. A second peak occurs after 50 years related to Paget's osteosarcoma. *Parosteal osteosarcoma* is rare, but regarded as a distinct sub-type and presents in the 20–40 age group. As a group the prognosis is better. In keeping with this, pulmonary metastases are not usually detectable at presentation, though may be apparent after a long symptom-free interval following incomplete excision. Some authors recognize further sub-types of juxtacortical osteosarcoma

(periosteal and surface osteosarcoma) (**REF: R122**). Although plain films allow assessment of peripheral bone involvement, computed tomography and magnetic resonance imaging are the only methods available permitting study of intramedullary extension prior to local resection. Similarly, soft tissue extension is demonstrated by CT, although appearances may be misleading in the presence of oedema or haemorrhage (e.g. after biopsy). CT is also useful to assess the presence of pulmonary secondaries.

Although multifocal osteosarcoma in bone does rarely occur, it is probably that most cases are due to bony metastases. Bone scintigraphy may reveal distant bone metastases or 'skip' metastases in the bone primarily involved.
**REF: R123**

A81    a *False*    b *True*    c *False*    d *False*    e *True*
     a    See notes following **A82**.
     b    See notes following **A83**.
     c    See notes following **A55**.
     d    Hypophosphataemia occurs in primary hyperparathyroidism.
     e    See notes following **A55**, **A56** and **A94**.

A82    a *False*    b *True*    c *False*    d *True*    e *False*

*Causes of hypercalcaemia*
1    Hyperparathyroidism — primary and tertiary, but not secondary.
2    Malignancy — basic mechanisms:
(a) Osteolytic metastases, e.g. carcinoma of the breast.
(b) Ectopic parathormone, e.g. squamous carcinoma of the lung.
(c) Parathormone-like substances.
(d) Multiple myeloma.
3    Sarcoidosis.
4    Drugs — hypervitaminosis D; milk-alkali syndrome.
5    Thyrotoxicosis — but rarely significant.
6    Adrenal insufficiency.
7    Idiopathic hypercalcaemia of infancy.
8    Prolonged immobilization (especially in Paget's disease).
**REF: R79**

## Locomotor System

**A83** a *True* b *True* c *True* d *False* e *False*

*Causes of osteomalacia/rickets*
1. Nutritional.
2. Malabsorption, e.g. coeliac disease, biliary atresia.
3. Renal disease.
   (a) renal glomerular failure: osteodystrophy; dialysis bone disease.
   (b) renal tubular disorders: familial hypophosphataemic rickets (hyperphosphaturia); adult onset hypophosphataemic osteomalacia (e.g. non-endocrine soft tissue tumours; giant cell tumour; neurofibromatosis; fibrous dysplasia).
   (c) renal tubular acidosis: inherited (distal type); acquired — ureterocolic anastomosis.
   (d) multiple renal tubular defects (Fanconi): cystinosis; Wilson's. cadmium poisoning.
4. Anticonvulsants.
5. Tumour rickets.
6. Vitamin D dependent.

**REF: R100, R124**

**A84** a *False* b *True* c *True* d *True* e *False*
Definition of *osteoporosis:* reduced bone mass of normal composition on histology.

*Classification*
1. *Idiopathic.* Post-menopausal; senile; juvenile; idiopathic.
2. *Endocrine/metabolic.* Hypogonadism; Cushing's; thyrotoxic; hypopituitarism; scurvy; chronic renal failure (as part of osteodystrophy); acromegaly.
3. *Immobilization.*
4. *Genetic.* Turner's; osteogenesis imperfecta; homocystinuria.
5. *Drugs.* Corticosteroids; heparin; cytotoxics.
6. *Others.* Chronic liver disease; coeliac disease; post-gastrectomy. (All three also cause osteomalacia.)

**REF: R100**

**A85** a *False* b *False* c *True* d *True* e *True*
Imaging is performed 2–4 hours after injection of the radionuclide. Although bone scintigrams are extremely sensitive in the detection of localized skeletal abnormalities, they are usually non-specific as to the cause.

## Answers and Notes

Hypertrophic osteoarthropathy gives a characteristic appearance of abnormal linear accumulations of radionuclide along the cortical margins of the tubular bones and, often, periarticular uptake due to synovitis (**REF: R125**). In the presence of an active inflammatory arthritis there is increased uptake of technetium phosphate due to hyperaemia (related to synovitis) and to the accompanying bone involvement.

*Causes of extraosseous uptake of phosphate bone agents*
These include:
1 *Physiological*. Renal, cartilage, normal and lactating breast.
2 *Artefact*. Injection site; free pertechnetate (stomach, thyroid).
3 *Pathological*. Areas of dystrophic calcification; heterotopic bone; infarcts (myocardial, cerebral); cellulitis; inflammatory arthritis; fluid collections (ascites, pleural effusions); pulmonary ossification; osteosarcoma metastases; various breast diseases (including primary carcinoma, fibrocystic disease), etc.
**REF: R126, R127**

A86 a *True*  b *False*  c *True*  d *True*  e *False*
Triad — oral and genital ulcers and eye inflammation. Other manifestations:
1 Peripheral arthritis clinically (about 50%), but no X-ray changes.
2 Sacroiliitis, occasionally with spondylitis. Probably no association with HLA-B27.
3 Enthesopathy (calcaneal spurs); thrombophlebitis and arterial thrombosis (including pulmonary arteries); CNS involvement (25%); skin lesions; colitis (ulcerative, but uncommon); fever.
**REF: R128, R82**

A87 a *False*  b *False*  c *True*  d *True*  e *False*
There is much geographical variation with marked differences over quite short distances. Prevalence tends to be higher in Anglo-Saxons especially in Northern Europe. Commonest in pelvis, followed by lumbar spine, upper femora and skull.

*Complications*
1 Pathological fracture, especially of upper femora and compression fractures of vertebrae.
2 Incremental fractures are seen on the *convex* borders of bowed long bones (cf., Looser's zones).

## Locomotor System

3 Malignant change — especially osteosarcoma but also fibrosarcoma, chondrosarcoma and rarely other sarcomas.
4 Spinal cord compression — at any level due to vertebral involvement, but also cervical level due to basilar invagination.
5 Ureteric colic is related to hypercalcaemia and hypercalciuria, especially with immobilization.
6 'High output' cardiac failure (with extensive disease) often quoted but extremely rare.

The three radiological phases of Paget's disease are: (i) active or lytic; (ii) combined lytic/sclerotic; (iii) sclerotic/reparative — correspond to the resorption and new bone formation seen histologically. The active phase is hypervascular, hence the enlarged meningeal vascular grooves.
**REF: R129, R130**

A88    a *False*   b *True*   c *True*   d *True*   e *False*
'Pigeon-chest' (pectus carinatum) is associated with rickets.
The conditions which predispose to *slipped femoral capital epiphysis* include:
1 Trauma (a history of a definite episode is infrequently obtained).
2 A rapid growth spurt (hence the peak age incidence, which is earlier in girls than boys).
3 Obesity; mechanical stress.
4 Rickets.
5 Hypothyroidism.
6 Renal osteodystrophy.
The epiphysis displaces posteromedially.
See also notes to **A59**
Osteochondritis of the femoral epiphysis may follow attempts at reduction of congenital dislocation of the hip, but in addition there is a true association of congenital dislocation of the hip and Perthe's disease.
Agenesis of the lower spine (caudal regression syndrome) is the most specific congenital anomaly associated with maternal diabetes. A spectrum of abnormalities is seen — from minor coccygeal defects to absence of segments below the mid-thoracic level. Sacral agenesis is the commonest.
**REF: R131, R88**

A89    a *True*   b *True*   c *False*   d *True*   e *True*
*Main causes of transverse metaphyseal lucencies in children/infants*

1 Normal variant in neonate.
2 Transplacental infections (e.g. rubella, syphilis*).
3 Leukaemia.
4 Neuroblastoma secondaries.
5 Haemolytic disease of newborn.
6 Scurvy*.
7 Systemic illness or stress in infancy or *in utero*.

* with increased width of zone of provisional calcification.

REF: R88

A90  a *False*  b *True*  c *False*  d *True*  e *False*

There are many causes of generalized or widespread increase in bone density, but the more important are as follows:
1 *Acquired — neoplastic*.
(a) Multiple osteoblastic metastases (breast, prostate).
(b) Myelofibrosis (myelosclerosis) — 50% of patients develop osteosclerosis. Sometimes mixed sclerosis and lysis; occasionally lysis. *Marked splenomegaly*; extramedullary haemopoesis; raised serum uric acid and secondary gout.
(c) Lymphoma.
(d) Multiple myeloma (monoclonal gammopathy)—rare variant.
2 *Acquired — metabolic*, etc.
(a) Paget's disease.
(b) Fluorosis — associated with osteophytes at the entheses and periosteal proliferation.
(c) Renal osteodystrophy.
3 *Congenital/inherited*.
(a) Osteopetrosis (manifestations may include *otosclerosis*).
(b) Pyknodysostosis.
(c) Diaphyseal dysplasias (= Engelmann's),
(d) Mastocytosis.
REF: R88, R132

A91  a *True*  b *True*  c *False*  d *True*  e *False*

*Causes of localized accelerated skeletal maturation*
1 Juvenile chronic arthritis.
2 Haemophilia.
3 Chronic infection e.g. tuberculosis.
4 Healing fractures.
5 Arteriovenous fistula.
Note that the first three causes may be grouped under the 'hyperaemic joint syndrome' (see **A57**). Synovioma is rapidly

Locomotor System 105

progressive and destructive and usually occurs after epiphyseal closure.
**REF: R88**

A92  a *True*  b *True*  c *True*  d *False*  e *True*

*Causes of rib destruction with a soft tissue mass*
1 Bone sarcoma — osteo-, chondro-, fibrosarcoma, Ewing's.
2 Metastasis.
3 Myeloma/plasmacytoma.
4 Lymphoma.
5 Pleural based tumour eroding rib, e.g. mesothelioma, metastasis, carcinoma of bronchus.
6 Osteomyelitis, including tuberculosis, actinomycosis, fungus.
7 Others — benign bone tumours (aneursymal bone cyst, giant cell tumour), Brown tumour, histiocytosis X, neurogenic tumour, thalassaemia with extramedullary haemopoiesis.

A93  a *True*  b *False*  c *True*  d *False*  e *False*
Causes of pseudoarthroses in the limbs include: congenital; osteogenesis imperfecta, fibrous dysplasia; neurofibromatosis; non-union after fracture.
**REF: R88**

A94  a *True*  b *True*  c *False*  d *False*  e *True*

*Soft tissue calcification*
1 *Metastatic* — high circulatory calcium or phosphate. Hyperparathyroidism and other causes of chronic hypercalcaemia; renal failure; hypo- and pseudo-hypo-parathyroidism.
2 *Calcinosis* — skin, subcutaneous tissue and connective tissue. Normal calcium metabolism: dermatomyositis (universalis, circumscripta); scleroderma/CREST syndrome; tumoral calcinosis (idiopathic hyperphosphataemia); idiopathic.
3 *Dystrophic* — calcification in damaged tissue without generalized metabolic disturbances. Multiple causes: e.g. neuropathic; post-infective; degenerative (vascular in diabetes mellitus, atherosclerosis); post-traumatic; neoplastic; miscellaneous — pseudoxanthoma elasticum, Ehler's-Danlos.
**REF: R100**

**A95** **a** *True* **b** *True* **c** *True* **d** *True* **e** *False*
Causes of heel-pad thickening: acromegaly; obesity; myxodema; thyroid acropachy; generalized peripheral oedema; phenytoin treatment.
**REF: R133, R134**

# Genitourinary Tract

**A96**  a *True*  b *False*  c *False*  d *True*  e *True*
See **A97**

**A97**  a *True*  b *False*  c *False*  d *False*  e *False*
Nephrocalcinosis is renal parenchymal calcification.

*Classification*
1  REGULAR CALCIFICATION
(a) *Cortex*
   Acute cortical necrosis
   Chronic glomerulonephritis (rarely)
   Chronic transplant rejection
(b) *Medulla*
   Medullary sponge kidney
   Hyperparathyroidism
   Renal tubular acidosis (primary, distal loop variety)
   Renal papillary necrosis
   Hyperoxaluria (primary and acquired) — also cortical, or diffuse
   Others — including causes of chronic hypercalcaemia
Causes of medullary calcification are also associated with renal calculi formation.
2  *Irregular Calcification* (Tissue damage). Tuberculosis, hydatid, renal carcinoma, amyloid.
**REF: R135, R136**

**A98**  a *True*  b *False*  c *False*  d *False*  e *True*
Although vomiting (from gastroenteritis, for example) can lead to uraemia, due to dehydration (pre-renal failure), the anaemia would point to a chronic cause of uraemia. The vomiting is likely to be secondary to the uraemia. The commonest cause of chronic renal failure in a woman of this age is chronic pyelonephritis. Bladder outflow obstruction would be very unusual in a patient of this age and sex, but obstruction, particularly of both ureters (retroperitoneal tumour or fibrosis),

i.e. post-renal failure, needs to be excluded. Renal papillary necrosis, due either to chronic analgesic abuse or sickle cell disease (note that the patient is black) is also a likely possibility.

**A99**  a *True*  b *True*  c *False*  d *False*  e *True*

Initial radiographs on admission of a patient in renal failure should include:
(a) Chest film: Fluid overload, Goodpasture's syndrome, cardiac size, renal osteodystrophy, intercurrent pneumonia.
(b) Abdomen: Renal calculi, nephrocalcinosis, tuberculosis and bilharzia, renal outlines.
(c) Hands: Hyperparathyroidism

The specific questions to be answered are:
(a) What size are the kidneys?
(b) Are they obstructed?
(c) What is the cause of the renal failure?

Ultrasound examination can answer the first two questions without recourse to early high-dose intravenous urogram which is potentially hazardous. Information may also be gained as to the smoothness or otherwise of the renal outlines and, in some cases, (e.g. polycystic kidneys) clues to the aetiology. A later IVU may be necessary for specific diagnosis, e.g. chronic pyelonephritis (see **A100**).

**A100**  a *False*  b *True*  c *True*  d *False*  e *False*

*Diagnostic patterns on intravenous urogram in chronic renal failure*
Analysis of small kidneys
1  Small kidney with normal architecture — chronic glomerulonephritis, renal artery stenosis, atypical post-obstructive atrophy.
2  Small kidney with uniform papillary deformities and even parenchymal thinning — post obstructive atrophy, renal papillary necrosis (late).
3  Small kidney with irregular papillary deformity and uneven cortical thinning — chronic pyelonephritis, renal papillary necrosis, tuberculosis, multiple infarcts (calcyeal changes are often minor, but clubbing can occur).
**REF: R137**

**A101**  a *False*  b *True*  c *False*  d *True*  e *False*

*Renal papillary necrosis*

# Genitourinary Tract

*Causes*
Commonest:
(a) Chronic analgesic abuse.
(b) Diabetes mellitus.
(c) Sickle cell disease.
Others include:
(d) Obstruction with infection.
(e) Hypoxia and dehydration in infants.
(f) Acute suppurative pyelonephritis.
(g) Chronic transplant rejection.
(h) Alcoholism.
(i) Renal vein thrombosis.
*RPN may be present with:*
(a) Haematuria; flank pain and fever.
(b) Chronic renal failure.
(c) Acute renal failure with oliguria or anuria (due to sloughing of papillae and bilateral ureteric obstruction);
(d) renal colic.
(e) hypertension.
*Urographic appearances:*
(a) Total papillary sloughing — smooth clubbed calyces.
(b) Partial sloughing — papillary cavities, sinuses.
(c) Necrosis-*in-situ* — relatively normal or nephro-calcinosis.
*Renal outlines:*
(a) Usually smooth, but occasionally irregular outlines if long-standing (due to scarring between calyces).
(b) +/− Hypertrophy of columns of Bertin.
**REF: R138**

**A102**   a *True*   b *True*   c *True*   d *False*   e *False*
*Duplication anomalies* are often asymptomatic and vary from a split pelvis, to merging of the ureters at any point along their course or separate terminations in or outside the bladder. The most significant associations leading to secondary disease are:
(a) maldevelopment of the ureterovesical junction valve mechanism;
(b) ectopic ureteric orifice;
(c) ureterocele.
In the vast majority of cases the ureteric orifice draining the upper moiety is inferior and medial to that of the lower moiety. The upper moiety ureteric orifice may have an ectopic site in or outside the bladder, sometimes with a ureterocele. Non-function is usually found only in the upper renal moiety and is most frequently caused by obstruction with or without a

ureterocele and sometimes reflux. However, the lower moiety ureter is more prone to vesico-ureteric reflux.

There is a 50% incidence of multiple renal arteries to duplex kidneys (normal 25%). Secondary complications include: chronic pyelonephritis; stone formation and transitional cell carcinoma. Other associated anomalies include: atresia and congenital stricture of the ureter; rotation of the kidney.
**REF: R139**

**A103**    a *True*    b *True*    c *True*    d *False*    e *True*

The ultrasound appearance of the kidney itself in renal vein thrombosis (RVT) is non-specific, but thrombus may be seen in renal vein or vena cava. (**REF: R140**). Findings on the intravenous urogram are variable. In early RVT 25% have a normal intravenous urogram, but the kidney may be enlarged and the calyces compressed by oedema and renal function is diminished. The nephrogram may be normal, poor and persistent, or increasing in density. A sudden RVT may result in a large non-functioning kidney. In the more chronic phase the kidney may be normal in size or small with normal renal excretion.

Collateral venous channels may cause ureteral notching. RVT is a complication of underlying renal disease in the majority of adults, usually a membraneous glomerulonephritis, possibly related to a hypercoagulability state. Associations include:

1 Membraneous (or membrano-proliferative) glomerulonephritis.
(a) Often with nephrotic syndrome.
(b) 30–50% of these patients develop RVT.
(c) Underlying causes include SLE, drugs, diabetes, amyloid.
2 Transplant rejection.
3 Trauma.
4 Tumour.
(a) Extension of renal carcinoma.
(b) Local compression of vein by nodes, tumour.
5 Sickle cell anaemia.
6 Other hypercoagulability states, e.g. polycythaemia.
7 Idiopathic.
8 Infants.
(a) Dehydration.
(b) Infants of diabetic mothers.
**REF: R141**

## Genitourinary Tract 111

**A104** a *True* b *True* c *True* d *True* e *False*

Four major types of calculi

| Type | Frequency | Radiodensity |
|---|---|---|
| Calcium stones<br>Ca phosphate<br>Ca oxalate/phosphate<br>Ca oxalate | 70–80% | most dense |
| Struvite<br>(Triple phosphate/matrix) | 15–20% | less dense |
| Cystine | 1–3% | least dense |
| Uric acid | 5–10% | lucent unless<br>epitaxis (see below) |

Cystine stones are associated with homozygous cystinuria and contain sulphur, making them slightly radio-opaque. Uric acid lithiasis is not necessarily associated with hyperuricaemia. Struvite (magnesium ammonium calcium phosphate) calculi are invariably associated with infection with urea-splitting organisms, usually Proteus species.

*Major causes of calcium urolithiasis*
1 *Disordered calcium metabolism*
(a) Hypercalciuria with hypercalcaemia, e.g. primary hyperparathyroidism; sarcoidosis; malignant neoplasm; Paget's disease; immobilization; adrenal insufficiency.
(b) Hypercalciuria without hypercalcaemia, e.g. idiopathic; renal tubular acidosis (distal type); sarcoidosis; malignant neoplasms; immobilization; Paget's disease; Cushing's syndrome; medullary sponge kidney.
2 *Disordered oxalate metabolism*
(a) Primary oxaluria
(b) Acquired oxaluria, e.g. ileal disease or resection (but not ileostomy — see **A17**); malabsorption; jejunal bypass surgery.
3 *Calcium oxalate stones associated with hyperuricosuria*. Calcium oxalate crystals may be deposited on the surface of uric acid crystals (epitaxis).
4 *Idiopathic calcium urolithiasis*. Without hypercalciuria. Familial factors (e.g. lack of crystallization inhibitors) and environmental factors are probably important.
5 *Other factors affecting urinary saturation*, pH, etc, e.g. low fluid intake; dehydration (such as in chronic diarrhoea in ulcerative colitis); dietary intake.
**REF: R142**

**A105** a *True* b *False* c *False* d *False* e *False*

Although frank haematuria, flank pain and a palpable mass constitute the classic triad of clinical features in *renal cell carcinoma*, this combination occurs relatively infrequently. Systemic features occur in about 50%. These include weakness, weight loss, intermittent fever and anaemia. Occasionally there is erythrocytosis due to erythropoietin release from the tumour. Ectopic hormone production includes parathormone, prostaglandins, prolactin, renin, gonadotrophins and glucocorticoids. Reversible liver dysfunction is sometimes apparent, the cause for which is uncertain.

Seeding to the bladder is not a recognized feature; this does occur in transitional carcinomas.

Analgesic abuse is associated with an increased risk of transitional cell carcinoma (see **A108**). Computed tomography, when including a dynamic contrast-enhanced examination, is a highly accurate method of pre-operative staging of renal carcinoma. Assessment can then be made of the extent of local invasion, involvement of renal vein, inferior vena cava, and regional lymph nodes (example, **REF: R143**). Angiographic staging carries an error rate of up to 40%.

There is no increase in the prevalence of renal cell carcinoma in horseshoe kidney. However, transitional cell carcinoma is increased in this anomaly (see **A112**). Conditions that do predispose to renal cell carcinoma include von Hippel-Landau syndrome, and, probably, chronic haemodialysis.

**A106** a *True* b *True* c *True* d *False* e *False*

Berry aneurysms of the Circle of Willis occur in 10–15% of patients with adult polycystic kidney disease (**REF: R144**). Renovascular hypertension in *neurofibromatosis* occurs mainly in children and is usually related to renal artery stenosis. An adult with neurofibromatosis who develops hypertension is more likely to have a phaeochromocytoma. The stenosis is usually bilateral and proximal. There may be associated narrowing of the abdominal aorta. Occasionally mesenteric, coeliac, iliac and pulmonary artery stenoses occur. Histologically there is usually intimal and/or medial proliferation; less commonly there are intramural neurofibromas, or, possibly, tumours adjacent to the artery (**REF: R145**).

*Wilm's tumour.* This may be associated with congenital anomalies:
(a) Aniridia

(b) Hemihypertrophy — may precede or follow presentation of the tumour. May be ipsilateral or contralateral to the tumour.
(c) Wilm's tumour incidence also increased in: horseshoe kidney; crossed fused ectopia; hypospadias; cryptorchidism.
*Hemihypertrophy.* This is also associated with: medullary sponge kidney; Beckwith-Wiedemann syndrome; hamartoma; carcinoma of adrenal cortex; primary hepatic malignancies.

Renal hamartomas, also renal cysts, occur in *tuberous sclerosis.* NB: *von Hippel-Landau* syndrome is also associated with renal lesions (renal cysts, renal cell carcinoma) as well as retinal angioma, cerebellar haemangioblastoma (sometimes with polycythaemia), and phaeochromocytoma.

A107  a *True*  b *False*  c *True*  d *False*  e *False*

Comparison of features of *Wilm's tumour and neuroblastoma*

|  | Wilm's | Neuroblastoma |
|---|---|---|
| Age of presentation | Mostly <5 years rare <6 months | Sometimes infants Usually <3 years |
| Site | Intrarenal bilateral 5% | Sympathetic chain mostly adrenal |
| Affect on kidney | Enlarged Pelvicalyceal distortion | Displacement |
| Kidney function | Impaired more commonly | |
| Extension |  | More frequently crosses midline |
| Calcification | 5% | 50% metastase also calcify |
| Spread | Lungs IVC Liver | Paravertebral nodes Metastases to bone, skull sutures, liver |
| Associated abnormalities | Aniridia Hemihypertrophy Horse-shoe kidney | Catecholamine release VIP |

REF: R146

**A108** a *True* b *False* c *False* d *True* e *True*
Transitional carcinoma of the renal pelvis is uncommon (7% of all renal tumours). Peak age incidence is 50–70 years. Commoner in males than females overall. There is an association with chronic analgesic abuse; in this subgroup it is commoner in women.

The IVU findings are one of the following: discrete filling defects within the pyelogram; filling defects within dilated calyces; calyceal obliteration; hydronephrosis with renal enlargement; reduced renal function without renal enlargement.

Calcification is very rare (reported in only one series at 2%). Angiography is either normal or shows sparse malignant vessels and/or encasement (cf. most renal cell carcinomas which are hypervascular).

There is an increased incidence in the horse-shoe kidney (see **A112**) and other anomalies in which there is obstruction and infection.

Multiple tumours are frequent and there is a particular association with carcinoma of the bladder. This has given rise to the concept of the 'unstable urothelium' in certain patients **REF: R147**.

*Filling defects in the renal pelvis:*
(a) Calcidus.
(b) Tumour.
(c) Non-opaque blood clot.
(d) Pyeloureteritis cystica.
(e) Intramural haemorrhage.
(f) Vascular impressions (anomalous vessels, collateral arteries and veins).
(g) Infective material, e.g. fungus balls.
(h) Malakoplakia.
(i) Granulomas (TB, schistosomiasis).

**A109** a *True* b *True* c *False* d *False* e *False*
Radiological features of a perirenal abscess include:
1  Loss of definition of the (lower) renal outline.
2  Displacement and rotation of the kidney. The lower pole is displaced medially, superiorly and anteriorly. The kidney may appear larger due to radiographic magnification. The bulk of the abscess tends to lie posteriorly.
3  Loss of the upper segment of the psoas margin.
4  Extrinsic compression of the renal pelvis and proximal ureter.

# Genitourinary Tract

5 Fixation of the kidney with respiration.
6 Displacement of adjacent bowel. On the right the descending duodenum displaces medially and anteriorly, and the hepatic flexure displaces inferiorly. On the left the distal transverse colon displaces upward or downward, and the duodenojejunal flexure displaces medially.
7 Secondary signs, e.g. scoliosis (in <50%) concave to the affected side, diminished diphragmatic movement, pulmonary basal changes.
Infiltration of the flank stripe indicates extension beyond the perirenal space.
**REF: R20**

**A110** a *True* b *True* c *True* d *True* e *False*

*Causes of unilateral enlarged kidney (smooth or irregular)*
1 *'Physiological'*. Compensatory hypertrophy.
2 *Duplex kidney*. Only half are larger than opposite kidney.
3 *Crossed fused ectopia*.
4 *Neoplasm*. Primary and secondary.
5 *Cystic disease*.
(a) Multiple acquired cysts.
(b) Multicystic kidney (cystic kidney, atretic ureter +/− renal calcification).
(c) Adult polycystic kidney (unilateral enlargement in up to about 10%).
(d) Hydatid disease
6 *Obstructive hydronephrosis*.
7 *Inflammatory*.
(a) Acute pyelonephritis
(b) Xanthogranulomatous pyelonephritis (see **A115**).
8 *Trauma*. Oedema; haematoma.
9 *Vascular*. Renal vein thrombosis — acute stage.

Acute glomerulonephritis causes bilateral enlargement.

**A111** a *True* b *True* c *False* d *False* e *True*

*A classification of renal cysts (modified from Elkin)* **(REF: R148)***:*
1 *Renal dysplasia*.
For example:
(a) *multicystic kidney* (& focal variants). Non-functioning (in vast majority) with multiple cysts, sometimes calcification. Atretic

ureter. Unilateral, but associated with pelvi-ureteric junction obstruction on contralateral side.
(b) associated with lower urinary tract obstruction *in utero*.
**2** *Polycystic renal disease*.
(a) Adult type (autosomal dominant). Most manifest at 30–50 years (but may occur in childhood). Associated conditions: hepatic cysts (33%); pancreatic cysts (9%); occasionally cysts in lungs, spleen, ovaries, testes, epididymis, uterus and bladder. Intracranial berry aneurysms in about 15%. Possibly increased incidence of carcinoma of kidney.
(b) Newborn type. Renal failure develops soon after birth.
(c) Childhood type (recessive). Less severe renal involvement than above, but there is a spectrum between newborn and childhood types. Predominant clinical problem is hepatic fibrosis leading to hepatic failure or variceal bleeding.
**3** *Medullary cysts*.
(a) Medullary sponge kidney — (see **A114**).
(b) Medullary cystic disease (nephronophthisis). Causes chronic renal failure in first and second decade.
(c) Renal papillary necrosis (see **A101**).
(d) Calyceal diverticulum/cyst.
**4** *Simple renal cysts*. Single or multiple.
**5** *Multilocular renal cysts*. Rare, mostly childhood.
**6** *Miscellaneous*.
(a) Inflammatory. TB; associated with calculus; hydatid.
(b) Post traumatic (following haematoma).
(c) Associated with haemodialysis. Cysts frequently develop in the kidneys of patients on chronic haemodialysis (**REF: R149**). Neoplasms are also more frequent in these patients. There is also evidence that cysts develop in the native kidneys in patients receiving renal transplants.
(d) Trisomy syndromes.
(e) Tuberous sclerosis. Associated with hamartomas, but also cysts.
(f) von Hippel-Landau syndrome. Also increase in renal carcinoma.
(g) Beckwith-Wiedemann syndrome. (EMG syndrome — Exophthalmos, Macroglossia and Gigantism).
(h) Neoplastic (cystic degeneration in carcinoma).
**REF: R148, R150, R144**

**A112**  **a** *True*  **b** *False*  **c** *True*  **d** *False*  **e** *False*
*Horse-shoe kidney* is the commonest form of renal fusion. The

Genitourinary Tract            117

renal mass tends to lie at a lower level than normal, with the pelvis anterior or occasionally lateral. Fusion is between the lower poles in the vast majority but occasionally the upper poles are fused.
The anomaly predisposes to disease, namely:
1 related to urinary stasis due to obstruction at the pelviureteric junction. This is distinctly more common on the left. Consequences include infection, calculi, chronic pyelonephritis and transitional cell carcinoma of the renal pelvis;
2 abdominal aortic aneurysm above the level of the isthmus;
3 rupture through the isthmus due to abdominal trauma;
4 increased incidence of nephroblastoma (Wilm's tumour).
There is no increase in the incidence of renal cell carcinoma. Other co-existing congenital anomalies of the urogenital tract are fairly common.
The isthmus between the two renal masses usually contains functioning renal tissue.
REF: R151

A113  a *True*  b *True*  c *True*  d *True*  e *False*
Nephrotic syndrome is characterized by albuminuria, hypoalbuminaemia and oedema (and hyperlipidaemia).

*Causes of the nephrotic syndrome*
1 *Primary glomerular diseases*. e.g. systemic lupus erythematosus causes a membranous or membranoproliferative glomerulonephritis.
2 *Infections*. Post-streptococcal, hepatitis B, syphilis, leprosy, malaria etc.
3 *Drugs*. Gold, mercury, penicillamine.
4 *Neoplasms*. Lymphomas, leukaemia.
5 *Multisystem diseases*. Systemic lupus erythematosus, Goodpasture's syndrome, amyloidosis, etc. Sarcoid, Nail-Patella Syndr.
6 *Miscellaneous*. Diabetes mellitus, thyroid disease, chronic transplant rejection

A114  a *True*  b *False*  c *False*  d *False*  e *True*
Medullary Sponge Kidney (MSK) is due to ectasia of the distal collecting tubules in the renal pyramids.

*Clinical*
Usually middle-aged, M > F. Mild cases (the majority) are asymptomatic. Others are associated with recurrent kidney

infections, haematuria, renal pain, and ureteric colic. There is an increased incidence of ureteric calculi. One third have hypercalciuria. Most cases are uncomplicated and have normal renal function and blood chemistry. There is an association with hemihypertrophy. Changes are limited to the renal pyramids. Cysts at the apex of the pyramid vary in size and shape. The pathophysiology is obscure.

*Radiology*
The kidneys are normal in size or slightly enlarged. Early cases show no nephrocalcinosis. Medullary nephrocalcinosis may be indistinguishable from other causes on plain film, but in MSK calcifications are often cigar-shaped and not uniform in distribution. The hallmark of MSK on intravenous urogram (IVU) is the delineation by contrast medium of the ectatic, usually fusiform tubules which is seen as coarse streaking in the pyramids around radiopaque concretions when present. There may be papillary enlargement with splaying of the calyceal cups. The changes of MSK are usually bilateral, but may be unilateral or focal. Differentiation must be made from the normal papillary 'blush' seen commonly on high-dose IVU. In severe MSK, when there is superimposed renal infection, parenchymal destruction may be seen.

The IVU in patients with infantile polycystic disease can appear sponge-like, as it can in Beckwith-Wiedemann syndrome.
**REF: R148, R152**

**A115** **a** *False* **b** *False* **c** *True* **d** *True* **e** *True*
*Xanthogranulomatous pyelonephritis* (XPN) is a progressive infiltrating granulomatous reaction in which lipid-laden macrophage accumulation occurs in inflamed and often suppurating renal tissue. The most common associated organisms are *Proteus* and *E. coli*. It is usually a complication of obstruction, most often due to calculus. XPN may extend into perinephric tissue causing abscess formation, sinuses and fistulae.

The condition is commonest in adults. Typical presentation is with severe toxaemia, weight loss, anaemia, high erythrocyte sedimentation rate and fever.

*Radiology*
Often stag-horn calculus present. The kidney may be enlarged with an ill-defined outline due to oedema or infiltration. IVU usually shows no function in the affected kidney. XPN may clinically, radiologically and pathologically mimic renal cell

# Genitourinary Tract 119

carcinoma. Selective renal arteriography shows stretching of intrarenal branches and avascular zones, but sometimes there is neovascularity resembling carcinoma. However, the vessels contract to adrenaline (unlike carcinoma). Percutaneous biopsy is of little help and may spread infection. Surgical excision is the only effective treatment.
REF: R153

A116 a *True* b *True* c *True* d *False* e *False*

*Vesico-ureteric reflux* may be primary or secondary. Primary reflux tends to improve spontaneously as the child matures.

*Conditions associated with secondary vesico-ureteric reflux*
1 *Complete duplex collecting system.* Reflux usually into the lower moiety
2 *Ectopic ureter.* May or may not be part of a duplex system. Single ectopic ureter more common in boys. Bilateral ectopic ureters — 'absent bladder neck syndrome'.
3 *Posterior urethral valve or other outlet tract obstruction.*
4 *Prune Belly syndrome.*
5 *Neuropathic bladder.*
6 *Recent passage of ureteric calculus.*
7 *Primary magaureter.* Sometimes associated with Hirschprung's disease.
8 *Exstrophy of the bladder.*
9 *Transient reflux.* This is seen during an episode of cystitis (due to infection, radiotherapy or drug-induced).
10 *Other causes of interference with ureterovesical sphincter mechanism:* post-surgical; adjacent bladder diverticulum; TB; bilharzia; deroofed or ruptured cystocele. Para-ureteric hernia (a small saccule at the ureteric orifice) is a result rather than cause of reflux.
REF: R154

A117 a *True* b *False* c *True* d *False* e *False*

*Causes of retroperitoneal fibrosis (RPF)*
1 *Idiopathic.* 50–70%. Possibly an 'auto-immune' mechanism as there is an association with Reidel's thyroiditis, sclerosing cholangitis and orbital pseudotumour.
2 *Malignant disease.* Spread from pelvic carcinoma, carcinoma of the pancreas, retroperitoneal sarcoma, lymphoma, metastases from colonic and breast carcinoma. Carcinoid may

also cause RPF due to the intense fibrotic response to this tumour.
**3** *Drugs.* Methysergide (for migraine). Evidence against other drugs is largely anecdotal.
**4** *Inflammation.* Pancreatitis, diverticulitis, inflammatory bowel disease (particularly Crohn's disease).
**5** *Post-haemorrhage.* Traumatic, aortic aneurysm
**6** *Urinoma.*
**7** *Previous surgery and/or radiotherapy.*
**8** *Perianeurysmal/Periaortitis.* In addition to haemorrhage causing RPF, fibrous plaques are also seen around atheromatous or aneurysmal aortas. It has been proposed that this is an immune response to leakage of antigens from atherosclerotic plaques (**REF: R155**).

*Clinical*
Peak age incidence 40–60 years. Usually presents with loss of weight, anorexia, abdominal and back pain. Erythrocyte sedimentation rate is typically raised. Presentation may be acute with anuria due to complete ureteric obstruction.

Benign and malignant causes of RPF are often indistinguishable clinically, urographically, and at laparotomy — biopsy is necessary.

*Urographic features*
**1** *Bilateral hydronephrosis.* However, dilatation of the pelvicalyceal systems may be minor, reflecting the notion that the process may interfere with ureteric function rather than be primarily obstructive. This is also the reason stated for the ease with which the ureters may be retrogradely catheterized. May be unilateral at first (in up to one third).
**2** *Dilatation of ureters.* To level of obstruction (usually lower lumbar vertebrae).
**3** *Medial deviation of the ureters.* Not a useful sign. Ureters are often in a normal position.
**4** *Nephrogram.* Non-function, or persistent increasing or low density.
**REF: R156**

*Other radiographic signs*
Loss of psoas outlines is not a consistent finding. Occasionally there is obstruction or deviation of the aorta, IVC or iliac vessels. Duodenal and rectal encasement is also seen. Fibrosis may also extend into the mediastinum, porta hepatis, and

# Genitourinary Tract

mesentery. Rarely infiltration into the walls of hollow viscera has been reported.
CT and, to a lesser extent, ultrasonography are useful in delineating the lesion and its extent.
**REF: R157**

**A118**    **a** *True*    **b** *True*    **c** *True*    **d** *False*    **e** *True*
*Lateral compression of the bladder* ('tear-drop' or pear-shaped bladder) is seen in:
1 Pelvic haematoma.
2 Pelvic lipomatosis.
3 Retroperitoneal fibrosis (see **A117**).
4 Inferior vena cava obstruction — due to venous collaterals.
5 Lymphadenopathy (lymphoma or extensive carcinoma).
6 Lymphocele.
7 Normal variant — especially in Negro males. Probably due to iliopsoas muscle hypertrophy and a narrow pelvis (**REF: R158**).

Rarely multiple neurofibromatosis may cause bilateral compression deformity of the bladder.
**REF: R159** (See also **A120**)

**A119**    **a** *True*    **b** *True*    **c** *False*    **d** *False*    **e** *False*
Major causes of radiographically visible *bladder wall calcification* include:
1 *Schistosomiasis*. Linear, associated with calcification of distal ureter. Tends not to severely reduce bladder capacity.
2 *Tuberculosis*. Rare to produce bladder calcification. Most have renal lesions. Irregular calcification with severe reduction in capacity.
3 *Amyloidosis*.
4 *Neoplasm*. 0.5% demonstrate radiographically visible calcification.
5 *Alkaline encrusted cystitis*. Necrotic areas in cystitis in the presence of an alkaline urine may become encrusted with calcification which may be severe enough to be radiographically visible. This most commonly occurs in: cyclophosphamide cystitis; radiotherapy; *Proteus* infection.
    *Malacoplakia* ('soft plaques') occurs in bladder and elsewhere in the urinary tract and rarely the gastrointestinal tract. In the urinary tract it is usually associated with persistent infection. Subepithelial small (though reaching to 2.5 cm), soft masses

tend to involve the trigone and lower ureter. As they heal they appear umbilicated. Radiographically they are seen as smooth rounded filling defects most common at the bladder base.
REF: R160

**A120**   a *True*   b *True*   c *True*   d *False*   e *False*

Causes of medial placement of both ureters (i.e. overlying lumbar vertebral bodies):
1 Normal variant, especially in young male Negroes.
2 Iliopsoas muscle hypertrophy (lateral placement may also occur).
3 Abdominal and pelvic masses, e.g. lymph nodes.
4 Abdominoperineal resection.
5 Retroperitoneal fibrosis (but see **A117**).
6 Pelvic lipomatosis may cause deviation of the lower ureters, medially or laterally.
In the absence of signs of obstruction medial placement of the ureters is rarely significant.
REF: R161

**A121**   a *True*   b *True*   c *False*   d *False*   e *False*

*Causes of oligohydramnios*
1 *Urinary anomalies.*
(a) Renal agenesis (Potter's syndrome: bilateral renal agenesis, oligohydramnios, pulmonary hypoplasia and typical facies). Amniotic fluid plays a part in pulmonary maturation — hence association of oligohydramnios and pulmonary hypoplasia.
(b) Urethral atresia or valves.
2 *Growth retardation.*
3 *Post maturity.*
4 *Premature rupture of membranes.*

*Causes of polyhydramnios*
(Diagnosis should be reserved for the third trimester since apparent increases in fluid in the first and second trimester may be normal).
1 *Fetal.*
(a) CNS abnormalities — open neural tube defects (anencephaly, meningocele, myelomeningocele, encephalocele).
(b) Gastrointestinal obstruction — low level obstruction (e.g.

Genitourinary Tract 123

anal atresia) is usually accompanied by normal amniotic fluid volume.
(c) Congenital skeletal syndromes — OGI, thanatophoric dwarfism, arthrogryposis.
2 *Maternal.*
(a) Diabetes mellitus — more severe degrees of diabetes mellitus cause growth retardation and hence oligohydramnios.
(b) Iso-immunization.
3 *Placental.* Chorioangioma.
4 *Idiopathic.* Most common cause. Normal fetus and mother, but still subject to the complications of hydramnios; namely malpresentation, cord prolapse or entanglement, premature labour, abruptio placenta, uterine atony and post-partum haemorrhage.
**REF: R162, R163**

A122  a *False*  b *True*  c *False*  d *False*  e *False*
The fetal spine is clearly and easily delineated by ultrasound at 16–17 weeks gestation. In the transverse plane the two posterior and one anterior ossification centres surround the spinal cord in a triangular configuration. In spina bifida there is separation of the posterior centres on transverse scans (lines further apart than at levels above and below). Associations: encephalocele; hydrocephalus; Arnold-Chiari II malformation (**REF: R164**).

In the second and third trimester, close examination may reveal a single umbilical artery. There is a 30–50% chance of coexistent fetal anomaly — usually renal or cardiac.

The most characteristic ultrasound pattern of bowel obstruction in the fetus is the 'double bubble' sign of duodenal obstruction. Two cystic structures represent distended stomach and proximal duodenum. Hydramnios is present in 50%. The 'pseudo-double-bubble' sign is due to a normal stomach with a prominent incisura, giving rise to bubbles in proximal and distal parts of stomach (**REF: R165**).

*Causes of duodenal obstruction* — duodenal stenosis/atresia; congenital webs; extrinsic bands; annular pancreas. Association (present in nearly 50%): Down's syndrome; malrotation; congenital heart disease; tracheo-oesophageal fistula; renal malformation.

Inability to identify a normal cranial vault by 12–14 weeks is highly suggestive of anencephaly. Polyhydramnios is present in 40–50% but not usually present until 26 weeks gestation (**REF: R164**).

Physiological calcium deposition occurs to a varying degree in the near-term placenta. After 33 weeks 50% show calcification. This is recognizable on ultrasound examination. It is of no apparent clinical or pathological significance (**REF: R166**).

**A123**    **a** *False*    **b** *False*    **c** *True*    **d** *True*    **e** *True*

Fetal heart motion can be reliably detected by high-resolution real time or M-mode ultrasound after 7 weeks gestation. Gestational age may be assessed by the following methods according to the stage of pregnancy:
1   Crown-Rump length — 7th to 10th week.
2   Biparietal diameter (BPD) — accuracy maximal 12–28 weeks. After this the biological variation in BPD widens and a single BPD measurement is inaccurate in defining gestational age. In practice serial measurements at approximately 14 and 32 weeks may be made.
3   Other parameters include femur length which is accurate from 10–12 weeks to term (**REF: R167**). The basis for the diagnosis of intrauterine growth retardation (IUGR) is the correlation of gestational age with fetal size. Accurate methods ideally depend on the prior assessment of gestational age early in pregnancy. BPD measurement and its correlation to the previously known gestational age is insensitive due to relative sparing of the brain in IUGR. Measurement of the abdominal perimeter at the level of the liver is reported to be sensitive since this correlates with fetal weight. The ratio of head perimeter to abdominal perimeter has been used but is subject to inaccuracies due to the degree of brain sparing being variable. Sonographically estimated fetal weight derived from head and abdominal measurement may also be used (**REF: R168**).

A false diagnosis of *placenta previa* may be made when an overdistended bladder compresses the anterior myometrium against the posterior wall of the uterus. Conversely, underfilling may render it impossible to identify the relationship of the lower margin of a low-lying placenta to the internal os. The examination should therefore be performed with varying degrees of bladder filling. A diagnosis of placenta previa should be confirmed clinically and by later repeat ultrasound, since a low-lying placenta may migrate superiorly during the formation of the lower uterine segment (**REF: R166**).

A grossly enlarged placenta is associated with: maternal diabetes mellitus; maternal anaemia; rhesus incompatibility;

chronic intrauterine infection. The size of the placenta is assessed visually.
REF: R166

A124 a *True* b *True* c *True* d *False* e *False*
The association of ovarian benign, solid tumours — usually fibromas — and pleural effusion constitutes *Meig's syndrome*. The effusion is usually right-sided and there is also ascites; both undergo resolution on removal of the tumour. The exact cause of the pleural effusion is speculative, but the ascites is caused by leakage of fluid from the tumour. 'Pseudo-Meig's syndrome' is applied to the combination of peritoneal and pleural fluid with ovarian epithelial cysts, teratomas, cystadenocarcinomas and Krukenberg tumours, and uterine fibroids, in which the fluid also resolves on tumour excision (**REF: R169**).

Trophoblastic tumours include *hydatidiform* mole (which may be non-invasive or invasive) and choriocarcinoma. The latter is preceded by a mole in 50%, a normal pregnancy in 25% and abortion in 25%. Hydatidiform mole comprises an irregular mass of grape-like vesicles and it may follow normal pregnancy, abortion or ectopic pregnancy. Abortion occurs in most cases within a few weeks of conception. Ultrasound examination is the imaging method of choice in hydatidiform mole; it appears as a homogeneous vesicular intrauterine mass. Fetal parts are occasionally identified. Bilateral theca lutein cysts occur in 44%, and are related to the high circulating levels of gonadotrophins (**REF: R169, R170**).

*Endometriosis* is the presence of functioning endocrine tissue outside its normal site in the lining of the uterus. It occurs especially in nulliparous women, during the reproductive years. Most frequent symptoms are pelvic pain, dyspareunia, dysmenorrhoea, and secondary infertility. Extrapelvic deposits of endometrium occasionally occur, for instance in the pleura where catamenial pneumothorax may result.

Commonest sites include — ovaries, pouch of Douglas, peritoneal surface of uterus, fallopian tubes, posterior fornix of vagina, bladder, ureters, rectosigmoid, small intestine. Adhesions in the pelvis are a prominent feature of endometriosis resulting from haemorrhage.

Involvement of the rectosigmoid presents with constipation, diarrhoea and pain, but not rectal bleeding as the mucosa is intact. A transverse ridge ('shelf tumour') on the anterior wall of the rectum is typical, but strictures and polypoid masses also

occur. Small intestinal involvement is usually at the terminal ileum, and symptoms are related to obstruction from adhesions. Laparoscopy is the most useful study. Ultrasonography is non-specific, showing cystic, solid or complex masses difficult to distinguish from other adnexal masses (**REF: R169, R171**).
Carcinoma of the body of the uterus is more common in diabetics.

**A125**  a *False*  b *True*  c *False*  d *False*  e *False*

*Adenomyosis* (uterine endometriosis) consists of glandular tissue, with surrounding stroma, growing diffusely into uterine musculature. Quite often associated with fibroids. Presents usually with menorrhagia. Hysterosalpingography (HSG) — uterus usually enlarged, with short spicules extending outwards from uterine cavity for 1–4 mm, occasionally longer. In 30% of cases, projections terminate in rounded sacs, 2–4 mm in size. Normal variants which produce endometrial irregularity:
(a) Small cavities in uterine wall, especially in lower half of uterus. Adenomyosis found in only 25% of cases.
(b) Spiculated outline — due to gland filling in atrophic endometrium.

*Unicornuate uterus* is associated with a high incidence of urinary tract abnormalities, especially ipsilateral renal agenesis and renal ectopia. Lesser incidence of these findings in bicornuate uterus.

*Optimum time for HSG* is towards end of first week after menstrual period — isthmus is then at its most distensible and fallopian tubes are most easily filled. Pregnancy will not be present.

*Diverticulosis of the fallopian tubes.* HSG shows minute loculations up to 2 mm in diameter, usually on only proximal half of fallopian tubes clustered over a length of usually 1–2 cm. Inflammatory changes often found and co-existent tubal obstruction is a definite association. Diverticulosis is differentiated from tuberculosis, on HSG, by the consistent nodular appearance of the diverticula.

Features of *tuberculous salpingitis*:
1  Calcification in fallopian tubes, ovaries and regional lymph nodes.
2  Tubal occlusion in isthmus or ampulla is common; often absent or only slight dilatation.
3  Thickening of longitudinal mucosal folds.

# Genitourinary Tract

4 Small fistulae or irregular tubal recesses. Occasionally tubointestinal and tubovescical fistulae.
5 Rigid and straightened ('pipe stem') tube.
Fallopian tube calcification is not seen in diabetes, but calcification of uterine arteries sometimes occurs (**REF: R169**).

*Gynaecological calcifications*
1 *Uterine fibroids.* Post necrosis or post menopause. Usually 'sponge-like', occasionally peripheral only.
2 *Ovarian cystadenoma and cystadenocarcinoma.* Serous type may have psammoma body calcification — punctate and hazy. Metastases (peritoneum, liver, lymph nodes, lung) may calcify. Mucinous tumours occasionally cause pseudomyxoma peritonei, with fairly coarse calcification.
3 *Benign cystic teratomas of ovary* ('dermoid cysts'). Teeth in 30%, bone in 40%. Occasionally rim calcification, rarely homogeneous calcification (also have mottling due to mixture of sebum and hair).
4 *Malignant teratomas of ovary.* Occasional linear branching spicules of calcification. Recognizable teeth and bone are rare.
5 *Ovarian fibroma.* Stippled and mottled calcification secondary to necrosis.
6 *Ovarian thecoma.* Rarely fine, granular calcification.
7 *Gonadoblastoma.* Mottled or punctate calcification in 50%.
8 *Tuberculous salpingitis.* See above.

A126   a *True*   b *False*   c *True*   d *True*   e *True*

*Gynaecological causes of pneumoperitoneum*
1 Post abdominal surgery (usually disappears in one week, rarely 3).
2 Laparoscopy or tubal insufflation. Carbon dioxide absorbed in a few hours.
3 Vaginal douche with a bulb syringe or effervescent fluid.
4 Abnormal laxity of genital tract in postpartum period, especially when exercises in knee-elbow position. Similar mechanism in post menopausal women with patulous genital tract and prolapse.
5 Water ski-ing without wet suit.

*Complications of hysterectomy — radiological manifestations*
1 *Haematoma.* Usually between upper end of vaginal stump

and pelvic peritoneum. Seen in IVU and ultrasonography.
2  *Pelvis sepsis.* Risk in pelvic haematoma. Causes paralytic ileus and lack of definition of pelvic structures.
3  *Ureter.* Unusual after simple hysterectomy, common after radical hysterectomy. Due to direct operative trauma, especially where ureter crosses uterine vessels. Stripping of overlapping Waldeyer's sheath may endanger ureteral vascularity and nerve supply.
(a) Transient hydroureter and hydronephrosis.
(b) Stricture.
(c) Ureterovaginal fistula.
(d) Ureteral severance.
4  *Bladder.* Especially after radical hysterectomy.
(a) Vesicovaginal fistula.
(b) Postoperative bladder calculi.
(c) Urinary retention (denervation).
5  *Other complications.* e.g. deep vein thrombosis, paralytic ileus.
**REF: R169**

# Respiratory System

**A127** a *True* b *True* c *False* d *False* e *False*
*Emphysema* is permanent dilatation of air-spaces distal to the terminal bronchioles. There are two important types of emphysema, which may be combined: panlobular (or panacinar) (PLE); centrilobular (CLE).

*Centrilobular emphysema*
Coexists with chronic bronchitis in the UK. Therefore terms such as Chronic Obstructive Airways Disease are useful. Purer syndromes (emphysema without bronchitis) appear to be commoner in the USA.

*Panlobular emphysema*
May be associated with CLE and chronic bronchitis. Occurs in older patients ('emphysema of non-smokers'), but note association in younger patients with alpha-l-antitrypsin deficiency.

American texts (**REF: R172**) tend to recognize two main radiological patterns of altered pulmonary vascularity in emphysema, with a tendency to the clinical and pathological correlates as outlined below.
1 *Increased markings* (IM). Increased vascular shadows. Less severe overinflation. Pulmonary hypertension in most, cor pulmonale in many. Cardiac enlargement frequent. Bullae unusual.
2 *Arterial deficiency* (AD). Triad of peripheral oligaemia, overinflation, bullae. Hilar pulmonary artery enlargement (i.e. pulmonary hypertension) when this is generalized.

No absolute relationship but tendency is:
AD = PLE = pink puffers
IM = CLE = blue bloaters

|  | CLE | PLE |
|---|---|---|
| Clinical | Upper zone<br>Tend to be<br>'blue boaters'<br>Normal $O_2$, raised $CO_2$<br>Chronic bronchitis<br>Smokers | Random, some predilection for<br>lower zones<br>Tend to be<br>'pink puffers'<br>Normal gases at rest<br>Older patients<br>Also alpha-1 antitrypsin deficiency |
| Radiology | IM (but see below) | AD |

The existence of 'increased markings' type is contentious; in practice there is probably always a combination of chronic bronchitis and emphysema. In particular what is the relationship of the IM pattern (tending to be CLE) to the 'dirty chest' of chronic bronchitis in the UK? Possibly IM = chronic bronchitis + pulmonary hypertension. In reality it is not possible (or necessary) to separate the changes of chronic bronchitis and emphysema.
**REF: R173, R174**

**A128**  a *True*  b *False*  c *True*  d *False*  e *False*
See **A127**. Individuals homozygous for deficiency of this enzyme develop early panlobular, predominantly basal, emphysema. Some develop liver diseases, including neonatal hepatitis, childhood cirrhosis or cirrhosis in adulthood.
**REF: R175**

**A129**  a *True*  b *True*  c *True*  d *False*  e *False*

**Cystic fibrosis**

Autosomal recessive. Viscid mucus secretions lead predominantly to pancreatic dysfunction and chronic diffuse obstructive pulmonary disease.
1  *Neonatal meconium ileus*. Sometimes with volvulus, meconium peritonitis, or ileal atresia.
2  *Failure to thrive*. Malabsorption due to pancreatic insufficiency, recurrent chest infections and, sometimes, recurrent pancreatitis.

Respiratory System 131

3 *Children and young adults*. Small or large bowel obstruction — 'meconium ileus equivalent', intussusception, volvulus, rectal prolapse, rectal impaction. Liver — biliary cirrhosis leading to portal hypertension. Increased gall-stones. Infertility. Recurrent chest infections leading to bronchiectasis, abscesses, fibrosis, respiratory failure and cor pulmonale.

*Radiology*
1 *Chest*. Pattern of extensive small and medium airways obstruction — a 'dirty lung'. Bronchial wall thickening; mucus plugging; atelectasis; recurrent pneumonic consolidation (especially Staph. and Pseudomonas) and focal inflammatory infiltration; focal air trapping and thin-walled air-filled cysts; bronchiectasis; abscesses, 'shaggy heart sign'; pneumothorax. Later generalized hyperinflation, coarse fibrosis (honeycomb), cor pulmonale.
2 *Sinuses*. Evidence of chronic sinusitis. Polyps; mucoceles.
3 *Abdomen*. Signs of meconium ileus, obstruction, etc. (see above). Pancreatic calcification. Gall-stones. Later portal hypertension.
4 *Skeletal*. Hypertrophic pulmonary osteo-arthropathy; retarded maturation.
**REF: R176, R177**

A130 a *True* b *True* c *False* d *False* e *True*
*Bronchiectasis* — is irreversible dilatation of the bronchial tree. Tends to be local. In chronic bronchitis there is mild generalized bronchial dilatation, but chronic bronchitis and bronchiectasis often co-exist.

*Causes of bronchiectasis*
1 *Complications of childhood pneumonia*. Especially pertussis and measles.
2 *Chronic bronchial obstruction*.
(a) Arising from wall — adenoma.
(b) Congenital — Kartagener's bronchial cartilage abnormal, e.g. tracheomalacia.
(c) Lumen — foreign body.
(d) Mucus plugs: asthma; cystic fibrosis; allergic bronchopulmonary aspergillosis.
3 *Recurrent infections*: chronic aspiration; agammaglobulinaemia; chronic granulomatous disease of

childhood; infection of intralobar sequestration cyst.
4 *Complication of many primary lung disease*. e.g. part of Macleod's syndrome; fibrotic lung disease; tuberculosis.
**REF: R178**

A131  a *True*   b *False*   c *False*   d *False*   e *False*

**Sarcoidosis**
Most commonly affects young adults presenting with bilateral hilar lymphadenopathy, erythema nodosum and acute eye inflammation, often with fever. This mode of presentation has a good prognosis. A more insidious onset is seen in older patients, often with pulmonary parenchymal involvement at the time of presentation. Parenchymal lung disease completely resolves only in about 40% of patients.

*Changes on CXR*
1 *Lymph node enlargement*. Bilateral hilar lymph node enlargement (BHL). BHL + right paratracheal (Garland's triad). BHL + bilateral paratracheal. Occasionally unilateral hilar node enlargement (up to 5%). Anterior mediastinal nodes rarely affected (cf. lymphoma). Rarely calcification of lymph nodes — 'egg shell' (up to 5%).
2 *Parenchymal involvement*. A great mimic but commonest is mid-zone reticulo-nodular pattern. Atypically a chronic acinar pattern, localized extensive disease (segmental or lobar consolidation); bullae; bronchiectasis; later resolution or fibrosis (upper zone). Pneumothorax. Very rarely calcification of parenchymal lesions (not related to hypercalcaemia). Pleural effusion rare (about 2–5%).

*Heart*
Cardiomegaly — may be related to cardiomyopathy, cor pulmonale (secondary to fibrotic lung disease), heart block, pericardial effusion.

Gallium $^{67}$ citrate scintigraphy is a sensitive test for active sarcoid, but non-specific. A negative scintigram coupled with negative serum angiotensin converting enzyme estimation has a high predictive value for excluding active sarcoid.
**REF: R179 - R181**

Respiratory System    133

**A132**   a *False*   b *True*   c *False*   d *True*   e *True*

*Macleod's (or Swyer-James') syndrome* is now thought to be due to a (probably viral) lower respiratory tract infection in childhood causing acute bronchiolitis and resultant destructive changes in a way similar to panacinar emphysema. Pathologically there is bronchitis, bronchiolitis, bronchiolitis obliterans and emphysema.
Abnormality may affect one lung or one or more lobes.
Macleod's syndrome is a cause of *unilateral hyperlucency of a hemithorax*.
*Other causes of unilateral hyperlucency.*
(a) Radiographic — rotation.
(b) Chest wall: mastectomy; poliomyelitis; congenital absence of pectoralis major (Poland's syndrome).
(c) Spurious — increased density on contralateral side.
(d) Pneumothorax.
(e) Pulmonary causes: obstructive hyperinflation, e.g. inhaled foreign body; compensatory hyperinflation; unilateral massive pulmonary embolus; giant bullae; congenital lobar emphysema; pulmonary artery agenesis.
*Chest radiograph in Macleod's syndrome.*
(a) Hypertransradiancy of one lung (or lobe) due to decreased perfusion.
(b) Small peripheral pulmonary vessels.
(c) Ipsilateral hilum diminutive but present (cf. absence in unilateral pulmonary artery agenesis).
(d) In inspiration volume of affected lung equal to or smaller than normal lung, rarely larger (small lung in pulmonary artery agenesis).
(e) Air trapping in expiration (cf. no air trapping in pulmonary artery agenesis).
(f) Contralateral side may be plethoric.
*Pulmonary angiography.* Diminutive hilar vessels and attenuated peripheral vessels.
*Bronchography.* Irregular dilatation of segmental bronchi with termination at 5th–6th stage divisions.
**REF: R178**


**A133**   a *True*   b *False*   c *True*   d *False*   e *True*

*Drug induced pulmonary disease*
Five patterns:
1  *Diffuse interstitial* (reticulonodular).

## Answers and Notes

(a) Mainly *cytotoxics*. Busulphan, bleomycin, methotrexate, cyclophosphamide. Remember pneumocystis pneumonia and other opportunists in the differential diagnosis.
(b) Nitrofurantoin — chronic stage.
2 *Diffuse alveolar*. Include opiates, nitrofurantoin (acute), salicylates, amiodorone.
3 *Pleural effusion* or *Pleural fibrosis*. Mainly lupus erythematosus-like syndromes, e.g. hydralazine, procainamide. Methysergide; beta-blockers.
4 *Hilar enlargement or mediastinal enlargement*. Phenytoin, trimethadone (glandular); corticosteroids (fat).
5 *Localized consolidation*. Nitrofurantoin, penicillin, sulphonamides.

Adriamycin does not produce pulmonary disease in the absence of previous radiotherapy.

Previous administered cytotoxics may enhance the pulmonary toxicity of radiotherapy and vice versa (**REF: R182, R183**).

A134    a *False*    b *False*    c *True*    d *False*    e *True*
Bird Fancier's lung is one of the extrinsic allergic alveolitides (EAA). EAA's tend to cause lower zone changes in the acute phase and upper zone fibrosis with chronic exposure to the antigen. Pleural effusion is rare (**REF: R184, R185**).

*Causes of upper lobe fibrosis*
Tuberculosis
Sarcoid
Pneumoconiosis
Radiotherapy
EAA
Ankylosing spondylitis
Aspergillosis — chronic allergic bronchopulmonary
(Mnemonic: **A STREP A**)

The *aspergillus* fungus causes three types of pulmonary disease:
1 *Invasive aspergillosis*. Immunocompromised hosts.
Radiological appearances — rounded peripheral opacities, progressing to consolidation and cavitation. Widespread dissemination often occurs.
2 *Mycetoma*. Saprophytic colonization of a pre-existing cavity. Considered non-invasive but may be so in an immunocompromised host. Radiology — one or more rounded,

Respiratory System 135

mobile densities in a cavity (usually upper lobe).
3 *Allergic bronchopulmonary aspergillosis* (ABPA).
Asthma, blood eosinophilia, recurrent pulmonary densities, immediate skin reaction to antigen testing, serum precipitins, raised IgE. Radiology — bronchial wall thickening (commonest finding); segmental or lobar collapse; (perihilar) consolidation; mucoid impaction (band shadows, 'gloved fingers'); proximal bronchiectasis; upper lobe fibrosis.

Despite the existence of these three separate entities, there is overlap, and the pulmonary aspergilloses are best regarded as a spectrum of disease.
Eosinophilic pneumonia — see **A135**.
**REF: R186, R187**

**A135**  a *True*  b *False*  c *True*  d *True*  e *True*
*Pulmonary eosinophilia* — pulmonary infiltrates with blood eosinophilia. A classification of eosinophilic lung disease which is predominantly allergic/immunogenic:
1 *Specific aetiologies.*
(a) Drugs, e.g. Nitrofurantoin, salicylates, sulphonamides, penicillins.
(b) Parasites. Localized — related to passage of larval forms of primary intestinal helminths through the lungs, e.g. ascaris, strongyloides, hookworm, schistosomiasis. Diffuse — 'tropical pulmonary eosinophilia', due to hypersensitivity reaction to microfilarial species.
(c) Fungal. ABPA in asthmatics. A minority of patients with asthma pulmonary eosinophilia (APE) have no demonstrable cause for eosinophilia.
(d) Occupational. e.g. exposure to epoxy resins.
2 *Idiopathic.* Transient (Loeffler's syndrome); chronic ('chronic eosinophilic pneumonias').
3 *Associated with vasculitis.* Collagen vascular diseases — polyarteritis nodosa and its variants such as Churg-Strauss syndrome.

Hodgkin's disease does not fit into this classification of hypersensitivity lung disease but mild peripheral eosinophilia is not infrequent, especially in patients with pruritis and Hodgkin's can, of course, produce pulmonary infiltrates.
**REF: R185, R188**

**A136**  a *True*  b *False*  c *True*  d *False*  e *True*
*Berylliosis* is not a true pneumoconiosis but is more probably

related to a delayed hypersensitivity reaction. Acute radiological manifestations include a fulminant form (pulmonary oedema) and insidious form (diffuse pulmonary haziness and irregular patchy opacities). The commoner chronic form resembles sarcoid in its pulmonary radiological manifestations. Calcification of pulmonary nodules can occur (cf. sarcoid) (**REF: R189**).

Talc exposure, though radiologically similar to asbestos exposure, does not predispose to mesothelioma.

Acute inhalation of *cadmium* fumes causes delayed pulmonary oedema. Chronic exposure causes diffuse emphysema. Renal damage also occurs.

*Byssinosis* is a disease of cotton, flax and hemp workers. The clinical presentation is virtually pathognomonic — 'Monday morning dyspnoea', symptoms being related to bronchoconstriction. Chest radiography is normal. Long-term exposure causes a clinical (and radiological) picture identical to chronic bronchitis and emphysema.

The inhalation of many noxious gases and soluble aerosols can cause pulmonary oedema associated with normal microvascular pressure. These include the dioxides of nitrogen and sulphur, carbon monoxide, chlorine and phosgene.

**A137**  a *False*  b *True*  c *False*  d *False*  e *False*

*Caplan's syndrome* is the combination of rheumatoid pulmonary nodules (granulomas) and underlying pneumoconiosis — usually coal worker's, but also silicosis, and occasionally asbestosis.

*Asbestos exposure*
1  Pleural manifestation.
2  Combined pleural and parenchymal.
3  Parenchymal only (approximately 20%).

The pleural changes (plaques +/− calcification +/− generalized thickening) are parietal and often involve the diaphragmatic pleura. Benign pleural effusions do occur, though the presence of an effusion should raise the suspicion of development of mesothelioma.

The parenchymal changes (asbestosis) are predominantly basal but later may extend to upper zones. Shadowing is nodular, reticulonodular or reticular. The 'shaggy heart' sign is due to a combination of pleural and parenchymal involvement.

# Respiratory System 137

Asbestos exposure does not predispose to tuberculosis. There is a predisposition to mesothelioma (pleural and peritoneal), bronchogenic (usually adenocarcinoma) and upper gastrointestinal and laryngeal and ovarian carcinoma.
**REF: R190, R191**

A138  a *False*  b *True*  c *True*  d *False*  e *False*
The classical appearance of 'simple' *silicosis* is of multiple nodules 1–10 mm in diameter, well circumscribed, predominantly mid-zone, preceded or associated with a reticular pattern. Nodules are better defined and denser than in coal worker's pneumoconiosis. Hilar lymph node enlargement is relatively common. 'Egg-shell' calcification of lymph nodes occurs in about 5% — almost pathognomonic (seen occasionally in sarcoid). Calcification of nodules, previously thought infrequent, probably occurs in 20%. 'Complicated' pneumoconiosis usually affects upper lobes and consists of large opacities or conglomerate shadows which may develop to 'progressive massive fibrosis'. Conglomerations may cavitate without tuberculosis infection, although silicosis predisposes to tuberculosis.
**REF: R192**

A139  a *False*  b *False*  c *False*  d *True*  e *True*
Pneumonia due to *Pneumocystis carinii* occurs in immunocompromised hosts with humoral and/or T-cell deficiency, e.g. transplant recipients, patients with lymphoma due to the disease itself or to cytotoxic therapy, patients on cytotoxic therapy for leukaemia and solid cancers, and AIDS patients.

The organism is a protozoan which causes an interstitial pneumonia followed by an alveolar exudate. The majority of patients have a normal or near-normal (perihilar haze) CXR in the early stages of symptoms. Classic changes occurring later are diffuse perihilar infiltration/interstitial shadowing (including septal lines), often progressing to alveolar shadowing. Atypical appearances include unilateral or localized consolidation.

Diagnosis: sputum is positive in only 6% of cases. Biopsy (percutaneous, open or transbronchial) provides the accurate means of diagnosis, though transbronchial brushings may also be positive. Pneumocystis coexists with other infecting agents (e.g. CMV) in 25%.

Treatment: cotrimoxazole (Septrin) is the first drug of choice.
**REF: R193, R194**

Mnemonic for interstitial lung disease in the patient with a known neoplasm ('NOD')
N  Neoplasm itself (lymphomatous/leukaemic infiltration; lymphangitis carcinomatosa).
O  Opportunistic infection (e.g. pneumocystis; fungal).
D  Drugs reaction (see **A133**). Other, less frequent, causes include transfusion reaction, pulmonary haemorrhage.

**A140**  a *False*  b *False*  c *True*  d *False*  e *True*
Four main types of bronchial carcinoma:
1  *Squamous cell*. Most common. Usually central.
2  *Oat cell*. Central or peripheral, but characteristically a small peripheral lesion with large mediastinal/hilar glands.
3  *Undifferentiated*. This plus above two comprise 90%.
4  *Adenocarcinoma*. Usually peripheral. Occurs in non-smokers. Associated with interstitial pulmonary fibrosis — cryptogenic, systemic sclerosis.
Also alveolar cell carcinoma (see **A142**).

Hypertrophic pulmonary osteoarthropathy is associated with malignant lung tumours in over 90% — usually squamous carcinoma. Phrenic or recurrent laryngeal nerve paresis are among the contra-indications to attempted resection.

Influence of cell type on radiological pattern in bronchial carcinoma:
1  As the *sole* finding a hilar mass is commonest in oat cell and virtually non-existent in adenocarcinoma.
2  A mass > 4 cm is very unlikely to be oat cell.
3  Apical tumours are uncommon. When the sole finding they they are usually squamous cell.
4  Atelectasis strongly indicates squamous cell.
5  Mediastinal widening is usually due to spread from oat cell carcinoma.
**REF: R195, R178**

**A141**  a *True*  b *False*  c *False*  d *True*  e *True*

Features of bronchial 'adenomas'

A group of slowly growing malignant tumours:
(a) Carcinoids 90% — only rarely gives rise to carcinoid syndrome.
(b) Cylindromas (adenoid cystic carcinoma and mucoepidermoid carcinoma) 10%.
Average age of presentation around 40 years (i.e. younger than bronchogenic carcinoma).
90% are centrally placed in the lung.
Presentation:
(a) haemoptysis or
(b) recurrent bronchial obstruction producing recurrent infection and then bronchiectasis.
They are typically of 'dumb-bell' configuration, only a part of the tumour lying within the bronchial lumen; thus bronchoscopic removal is not practical.
REF: R196

A142 a *False* b *True* c *True* d *True* e *False*

*Bronchio-alveolar carcinoma*
Rarest form of primary lung carcinoma (about 2%). Presenting radiographic pattern:
(a) Nodule or mass — usually peripheral.
(b) Consolidation — localized or diffuse.
(c) Spreads through air spaces with mucus production and desmoplasia. Secondary radiographic signs include pleural retraction.
(d) Air bronchograms are frequent, explained by period of indolent growth and sparing of larger airways.
(e) Extrathoracic metastases are as common as in other types of lung carcinoma. Osteoblastic skeletal metastases may occur.
REF: R197

A143 a *False* b *True* c *True* d *False* e *False*
Pulmonary involvement with *lymphoma* is commoner in Hodgkin's disease and is rarely unaccompanied by mediastinal lymph node involvement. A parenchymal lesion in a newly diagnosed patient with Hodgkin's disease without mediastinal/hilar lymphadenopathy is unlikely to be due to the lymphoma itself. The parenchymal disease usually occurs by extension from nodes along bronchovascular lymphatics centrifugally. Patterns include a coarse reticulonodular

shadowing extending from the hilum, which may resemble lymphangitis carcinomatosa, and localized areas of consolidation involving segments or lobes without collapse and often demonstrating an air bronchogram. Subpleural masses are strongly suggestive of lymphoma. Parenchymal masses may cavitate without complicating infection. Bronchial compression by lymph nodes is rare, but bronchial occlusion can occur due to endobronchial disease.

In some patients, particularly those with non-Hodgkin's lymphoma, there may be a rapid evolution of parenchymal disease due to lymphomatous infiltration, sometimes over a few days. The appearances must be differentiated from pulmonary oedema or opportunistic infection (**REF: R198**). Remember the differential diagnosis of diffuse lung disease ('NOD') — disease due to the neoplasm, opportunistic infection, or drugs (see **A139**).
**REF: R199**

**A144**    **a** *True*    **b** *False*    **c** *True*    **d** *False*    **e** *False*
Occupational factors increasing the risk of *carcinoma of the bronchus* include: working in the chromate industry, nickel refining, asbestos exposure, haematite mining, uranium mining, and exposure to arsenic and beryllium. Cigarette smoking greatly increases the risk in exposed individuals. Carcinoma of the nose and nasal sinuses is increased in woodworkers in the furniture industry.

The skin signs with internal malignancy include: acanthosis nigricans (especially carcinoma of stomach, squamous carcinoma — including bronchial — and lymphoma); dermatomyositis; ichthyosis (especially lymphoma); pachydermoperiostitis and hypertrophic pulmonary osteoarthropathy (especially bronchial carcinoma).

See **A205** for ectopic hormones produced by non-endocrine tumours.

**A145**    **a** *True*    **b** *False*    **c** *False*    **d** *True*    **e** *True*
*Lymphangitis carcinomatosa* may be bilateral or unilateral. Unilateral disease is more commonly seen in carcinoma of the bronchus and breast. Neoplasms that most commonly give rise to lymphangitis carcinomatosa include: carcinoma of lung, breast, oesophagus and upper gastrointestinal tract, pancreas, larynx, thyroid and cervix. Note that lymphoma (lymphangitis lymphomatosa) gives an identical appearance.

Respiratory System 141

**A146** a *True* b *False* c *True* d *True* e *True*

*Kerley B lines*
Visible due to perilymphatic oedema or thickening (infiltration, deposition or fibrosis). For example:
1 *Oedema.* Left ventricular failure; mitral stenosis; interstitial pneumonia.
2 *Lymphatic obstruction/infiltrations.* Lymphangitis carcinomatosa or lymphomatosa; sarcoid.
3 *Perilymphatic fibrosis/depositions.* Pulmonary haemosiderosis; chronic mitral stenosis; pneumoconiosis.
**REF: R200, R201**

**A147** a *True* b *True* c *False* d *True* e *True*

*Causes of pulmonary arterial hypertension*
1 *Intrinsic lung disease.*
(a) Chronic obstructive airways disease.
(b) Diffuse pulmonary interstitial disease/fibrosis.
(c) Pulmonary vascular disease, e.g. thrombo-embolic, emboli of parasites (schistosomiasis) and metastases (e.g. chorionepithelioma); primary pulmonary hypertension.
2 *Malfunction of the chest bellows.*
(a) Severe kyphoscoliosis.
(b) Neuromuscular disease.
(c) Gross obesity (Pickwickian syndrome).
3 *Diminished ventilatory drive.* e.g. Ondine's curse.
4 *In congenital heart disease.* This results from elevation of pulmonary blood flow and/or resistance.
(Pressure = Flow × Resistance.) With left to right shunts there is overload of the pulmonary circulation; raised pulmonary vascular resistance may follow with resultant hypertension. (If the pressure on the right side of the heart exceeds the left, shunt reversal occurs — the Eisenmenger syndrome.)
5 *Secondary to chronic pulmonary venous hypertension* (reactive pulmonary hypertension). This results from backward transmission of elevated left atrial or pulmonary vein pressure, e.g. in mitral stenosis. Reactive vasomotor and obliterative changes in the pulmonary vascular bed contribute.

*Cor pulmonale*
Definition — hypertrophy of the right ventricle secondary to malfunctioning lungs. Pulmonary hypertension is a prerequisite. 1, 2 and 3 are causes.

**A148** a *False* b *True* c *False* d *True* e *True*

Perfusion scintigraphy alone (without a ventilation study) is sensitive for the diagnosis of pulmonary embolism (PE) but non-specific (see below). However, a normal perfusion study is extremely rarely associated with PE. Ventilation/perfusion (V/Q) mismatching is associated with PE but in recent years the concept of probabilities has been applied to the interpretation depending on the relative size and number of defects demonstrated (**REF:** e.g. **R202**).

*Causes of abnormal perfusion scintigram other than PE*
1 *Lung disease.* Nearly all pulmonary diseases, e.g. neoplasm, infection, chronic obstructive airways disease.
2 *Cardiomegaly.* Left lower lobe perfusion defect.
3 *Skeletal abnormality.* E.g. Pectus excavatum; kyphoscoliosis.
4 *Prominent mediastinal structures.* E.g. tortuous aorta.
5 *Diaphragm.* E.g. paralysis, eventration.

*Causes of unilateral abnormal perfusion/normal ventilation other than PE*
1 Central compression of pulmonary arteries by: mediastinal/hilar tumours; fibrosis; node enlargement. (The vessels are easily compressed, whereas central airways are supported by cartilage rings.)
2 Vasculitis of pulmonary arteries.
3 Pulmonary artery agenesis.
**REF: R203**

Marked V/Q defects may be seen in acute asthma, particularly with mucus plugging.
For perfusion scintigraphy the radiopharmaceutical is best injected with the patient supine to allow even pulmonary distribution, but imaging should be in the upright position if possible for better visualization of the bases.
**REF: R204**

**A149** a *True* b *True* c *True* d *True* e *False*

*Factors that lead to pulmonary oedema*
1 Increased capillary hydrostatic pressure.
2 Increased capillary permeability.
3 1 and 2 combined.

4   Decreased plasma osmotic pressure.
5   Decreased lymphatic drainage.

*Causes of pulmonary oedema according to mechanism*
1   Increased capillary hydrostatic pressure.
(a) Left ventricular failure.
(b) Mitral stenosis.
(c) Pulmonary venous obstruction.
(d) Over-transfusion.
(e) Dysfunction of a papillary muscle after myocardial infarction leads to mitral regurgitation, pulmonary oedema, usually with little or no increase in heart size.
2   Increased capillary permeability.
(a) Toxic inhalation/ingestion, e.g. phosgene; metallic oxides; silo-filler's disease (oxides of nitrogen); smoke; aspiration of fluid — Mendelson's syndrome; drowning/near drowning; Paraquat.
(b) Immunological reaction, e.g. transfusion reaction; hypersensitivity pneumonitis.
(c) Drugs, e.g. nitrofurantoin; sulphonamides.
(d) Radiation injury.
(e) Heat stroke.
3   *Combination of 1 and 2/unknown*
(a) Adult respiratory distress syndrome: 'shock lung'; burns; sepsis; endotoxaemia; disseminated intravascular coagulation; trauma, etc.
(b) Renal failure.
(c) Fat embolus.
(d) Opiate overdosage.
(e) Neurogenic (e.g. brainstem haemorrhage, raised intracranial pressure).
(f) Rapid lung expansion following drainage of pleural effusion/pneumothorax.
(g) High altitude.
4   *Decreased plasma osmotic pressure.* Hypoalbuminaemia — renal, hepatic, nutritional causes and protein-losing enteropathy.
5   Lymphatic insufficiency.
**REF: R205**

A150   a *False*   b *True*   c *True*   d *False*   e *True*

*Unilateral pulmonary oedema*
Ipsilateral to the following conditions:

## Answers and Notes

1 Postural — prolonged lateral decubitus position.
2 Systemic pulmonary artery shunts for congenital heart disease.
3 Total bronchial obstruction — 'drowned' lung.
4 Unilateral aspiration — fresh or sea water, gastric juice, etc.
5 Unilateral veno-occlusive disease — congenital obstruction of venous return; obstruction by tumour.
6 Pulmonary contusion.
7 Rapid thoracocentesis of pleural effusion.
8 Rapid drainage of pneumothorax.

Contralateral to the following conditions:
(An area not perfused cannot become oedematous)
1 Congenital pulmonary artery hypoplasia.
2 Cardiac decompensation in a patient with Macleod's syndrome.
3 Pulmonary embolism.
4 Unilateral emphysema.
5 Lobectomy/pneumonectomy.
6 Pre-existing pleural effusion.
7 Unilateral sympathectomy.
**REF: R206**

**A151**  **a** *True*  **b** *False*  **c** *True*  **d** *True*  **e** *True*
Causes of *enlargement of the azygos vein*
1 Normally azygos vein enlarges in: inspiration (but note that maximally held inspiration is often accomplished by a Valsalva manoeuvre and hence a diminution in size); supine position.
2 Increased circulating blood volume, e.g. renal failure, overhydration, pregnancy.
3 Congestive heart failure.
4 SVC obstruction.
5 IVC obstruction.
6 Portal hypertension.
7 Constrictive pericarditis.
8 Pericardial effusion.
9 Total anomalous pulmonary venous return to azygous system.
10 Tricuspid regurgitation.

**A152**  **a** *True*  **b** *True*  **c** *False*  **d** *False*  **e** *True*
**a** See **A153**. It is suggested that delay in clearance of lung fluid is responsible and that vaginal delivery aids in this process. Onset

# Respiratory System 145

immediately after birth. Usually excellent prognosis. Chest film shows interstitial fluid, small pleural effusions and mild cardiac enlargement. Clears in up to 5 days.
**b** See **A153**.
**c** See **A153** for associations of neonatal pneumothorax.
**e** See **A153**. About one quarter of infants of diabetic mothers suffer HMD.

**A153** **a** *True* **b** *True* **c** *False* **d** *False* **e** *True*
*Meconium aspiration syndrome* classically occurs in post-mature babies. A chemical pneumonitis occurs as a result of plugging of the airways with meconium, which may act as a ball valve obstruction. Radiographically there are coarse widely-scattered areas of consolidation or under-aeration and areas of hyperinflation. The diaphragm is usually depressed. Distinction from pneumonia may be impossible. Prognosis is good, recovery usually occurring in 48 hours although radiographic clearing may take 1–2 weeks. Pneumomediastinum and/or pneumothorax occurs in 10–20%.

**Pulmonary and airway causes of neonatal respiratory problems** (excludes cardiac causes)

*Common*
**1** *Respiratory distress syndrome (hyaline membrane disease):* increased in prematurity; maternal diabetes; maternal chronic pyelonephritis; antepartum haemorrhage.
**2** *Transient tachypnoea of the newborn:* more common in term babies; caesarian section (hence diabetic mothers); breech deliveries.
**3** *Pneumothorax.* Asymptomatic in 1–2% of neonates.
*Predispositions:*
(a) positive pressure ventilation;
(b) assisted ventilation for pulmonary disease;
(c) meconium aspiration;
(d) respiratory distress syndrome;
(e) hypoplastic lung with Potter's syndrome and obstructive urological malformations;
(f) diaphragmatic hernia.
**4** *Meconium aspiration.*

*Uncommon*
**1** *Pneumonia.*
**2** *Pulmonary haemorrhage.* Usually in prematurity. Usually

associated with septic shock, disseminated intravascular coagulation, haemorrhagic pneumonia, dextran treatment for necrotizing enterocolitis or endotracheal tube manipulation.

3 *Pulmonary hypoplasia*. Associated with diaphragmatic hernia, Potter's syndrome (renal agenesis) and vertebral anomalies.

4 *Diaphragmatic hernia*. Usually left side.

5 *Tracheo-oesophageal fistula*. Associated defects are imperforate anus, duodenal atresia, gut malrotation, vertebral and rib anomalies, renal anomalies, ventricular septal defect and patent ductus arteriosus. 'VATER' association — ventricular septal defect, anorectal malformation, tracheal-oesophageal fistula, renal anomalies. Perhaps this should be VVATERR syndrome as vertebral anomalies (e.g. hemivertebrae, vertebral body hypoplasia, hypoplastic pedicles, scoliosis) and radial hypoplasia are also seen.

6 *Pulmonary dysmaturity* (Wilson-Mikity syndrome). Prematurity. Usually onset 1–4 weeks.

7 *Bronchopulmonary dysplasia*. Oxygen toxicity, usually follows hyaline membrane disease. Onset late in first week of life.

8 *Chronic pulmonary insufficiency of the premature*. Smaller premature infants. More chronic course than hyaline membrane disease. Also caused by deficiency of surfactin.

*Rare*

1 *Airway obstruction*. Choanal atresia; vascular rings; laryngeal web; etc.

2 *Pleural effusion*.

3 *Congenital lobar emphysema*.

4 *Intrathoracic mass*. e.g. Cystic adenomatoid malformation (note: may be radiopaque initially).

5 *Chest wall deformity*. e.g. asphyxiating thoracic dysplasia.

**REF: R207**

A154    a *False*    b *False*    c *False*    d *True*    e *True*

*Pulmonary sequestration* is a congenital anomaly consisting of a mass of dysplastic lung tissue with no normal connection to the tracheobronchial tree and pulmonary arteries. There are two forms — intralobar and extralobar.

|  | Intralobar | Extralobar |
|---|---|---|
| Pleural covering | Within normal visceral pleura | Completely separate pleural investment |
| Symptoms | Recurrent infection or incidental congestive cardiac failure due to shunting | As for intralobar |
| Sites | Above diaphragm | Above or below diaphragm |
|  | Lung bases L>R | Lung bases L>R |
| Arterial supply | Systemic (thoracic aorta) | Systemic |
| Venous | Pulmonary veins (usually) | Systemic |
| X-ray | Solid or cystic *Cavity +/− fluid level | Homogeneous mass |
| Associated anomalies |  | Diaphragmatic hernia Fistula to gastrointestinal tract |

*if infection occurs with drainage to bronchial tree.
Arteriography is helpful in pre-operative assessment.
**REF: R208**

**A155**  a *True*  b *True*  c *True*  d *True*  e *False*

*Causes of pulmonary cavitation*
1 *Inflammatory*. Pneumonia, especially Klebsiella, Staphylococcal, Pseudomonas. Pneumatoceles (air cysts) occur especially in Staph. pneumonia in children. Aspirational abscess — anaerobes. Tuberculosis. Fungal, e.g. aspergillosis, nocardia (blastomycosis, coccidiomycosis in USA). Haematogenous abscesses — septic emboli in drug abusers, (staph.), bacterial endocarditis, etc. Amoebic abscess. Hydatid after bronchial drainage. Granulomas, e.g. Wegener's, rheumatoid.
2 *Neoplastic*.
(a) Primary — any but usually squamous. Especially peripheral and upper lobe lesions. Thick-walled. Eccentric cavity. May be

intracavity body (tumour). May be thin walled in squamous lesions. NB. non-neoplastic abscess may occur distal to an obstructing neoplastic lesion.
(b) Metastatic — any but especially squamous carcinoma and sarcomas. Lymphoma.
3  *Trauma* — pulmonary contusion.
4  *Ischaemia* — cavitating pulmonary infarcts.
5  *Congenital* — following infection and bronchial drainage of: intralobar sequestration; bronchogenic cyst.
**REF: R178**

A156  a *False*  b *False*  c *True*  d *True*  e *False*

*Causes of intrapulmonary calcification*
These include
1  *Tuberculosis*. Active or inactive.
2  *Fungal*. Histoplasmosis, coccidiomycosis in USA.
3  *Varicella* pneumonia.
4  *Silicosis*.
5  *Lymphoma* — after treatment.
6  *Hamartoma* — about 30%. Classically 'popcorn' calcification.
7  *Metabolic* — e.g. hyperparathyroidism, especially renal failure.
8  *Amyloid*.
9  *Metastases*. Papillary and mucinous adenocarcinoma of thyroid, ovary and gastrointestinal tract; dystrophic calcification in necrotic metastases after therapy; sarcoma secondaries, especially osteogenic, chondrosarcoma (calcification or ossification).
10  *Broncholiths*.
11  *Pulmonary ossification* in mitral valve disease.
**REF: R209**

A157  a *False*  b *True*  c *False*  d *True*  e *True*
**Pulmonary hamartomas** may contain connective tissue, cartilage fat, smooth muscle and bone elements. They are usually discovered in patients over 40 years old. Radiographic appearance is of a solitary pulmonary nodule with sharp, often lobulated, borders. Multiple lesions are occasionally seen. Calcification is visible on plain radiography in about 30% ('popcorn' calcification is characteristic but variable patterns are seen). Cavitation is very rare. Growth is very slow and they are

Respiratory System 149

usually asymptomatic. Endobronchial hamartomas resulting in obstruction are very rare. CT may be useful in diagnosis, demonstrating fat within the lesion in 50%.
REF: R210

A158 a *True* b *True* c *True* d *False* e *False*

*Causes of pneumothorax*
1 *'Spontaneous'*. i.e. no trauma or overt underlying lung disease. Usually males 20–40 years, especially tall individuals, including Marfan's. Due to apical blebs, results from paraseptal emphysema.
2 *Traumatic*. Open or closed chest trauma. Iatrogenic.
3 *Underlying lung disease*.
(a) Chronic obstructive airways disease.
(b) Asthma.
(c) Chronic interstitial lung disease — especially Histiocytosis X (20–50%), also idiopathic pulmonary fibrosis, sarcoid, radiation pneumonitis, silicosis, tuberous sclerosis, lymphangiomyomatosis.
(d) Malignant neoplasms — especially sarcoma secondaries (mostly osteosarcoma).
(e) Pulmonary infection — infected infarct/abscess/septic embolus; tuberculosis.
(f) Other cavitating lung lesions — e.g. rheumatoid nodule; Wegener's granuloma; cavitating infarct; lymphoma.
4 *Neonatal pneumothorax* (see **A153**).
5 *Intrathoracic endometriosis* (catamenial pneumothorax).
6 *Oesophageal rupture*.
7 *Tracheobronchial rupture*.
8 *Diabetic ketoacidosis*.
9 *Secondary to any cause of pneumomediastinum*.
*Causes of pneumomediastinum:*
(a) May or may not be associated with pneumothorax — starts as interstitial emphysema due to increase intra-alveolar pressure and passes centrally and/or peripherally to pleural cavity and/or mediastinum. Following produce pneumomediastinum by this mechanism: (i) Valsalva manoevure, e.g. violent exercise, childbirth, coughing; (ii) recurrent vomiting, e.g. diabetic ketoacidosis; (iii) asthma; (iv) positive pressure ventilation.
(b) Oesophageal tears.
(c) Tracheobronchial tears.
(d) Extension of subcutaneous emphysema of the neck (paranasal sinus fractures).

(e) Tracheal trauma (tracheostomy, blunt trauma), transcricoid bronchography, etc.
(f) Extension of extraperitoneal gas.
Note that pneumomediastinum may also be associated with extension of air *to* the extraperitoneal spaces via the diaphragmatic hiatuses, and thence to the peritoneal space. Pneumomediastinum may also, of course, give rise to subcutaneous emphysema of the neck (**REF: R211**).
10  *Barotrauma* — (artificial ventilation).
11  *Pneumoperitoneum* — passage of air through a pleuroperitoneal foramen.
**REF: R212**

**A159**  a *False*  b *False*  c *False*  d *True*  e *False*

*Paratracheal lymph node enlargement*
1  *Infective.*
(a) Tuberculosis (primary).
(b) Fungal (histoplasmosis, coccidiomycosis).
(c) Infectious mononucleosis.
2  *Neoplasm.*
(a) Bronchogenic carcinoma.
(b) Other metastatic intrathoracic neoplasms, e.g. oesophagus. Extrathoracic — uncommon. Tumours of head and neck, genito-urinary (via thoracic duct), breast, melanomas (**REF: R213**).
(c) Lymphoma.
(d) Leukaemia.
3  *Inhalational.* Pneumoconiosis.
4  *Idiopathic.* Sarcoid; Histiocytosis X.

**A160**  a *False*  b *False*  c *False*  d *False*  e *True*
There is a marked variability in size and shape of the normal thymus. It is usually visible on chest radiography at birth and until 2 years or older.
  A small or absent thymus in infants (especially premature ones) is usually related to perinatal stress. Rebound enlargement may occur weeks to months after recovery.
Characteristics of a normal thymus on chest radiography:
1  'Notch' sign (indentation at the junction of thymic and heart shadows).
2  'Sail' sign (triangular density in the superior mediastinum, usually right-sided. 5% of infants).

3 'Wave' sign (undulation due to rib indentations).
4 Changes in respiration and position (more prominent in expiration).

The thymus is soft and even when large does not cause compression or displacement of adjacent structures.

*Thymic 'masses'*
1 *Neoplasms.*
(a) Thymomas — 20–35% malignant. 50% discovered incidentally. Associated systemic symptoms include myasthenia gravis, red cell aplasia, and hypogammaglobulinaemia. Myasthenia gravis is associated with thymic hyperplasia or thymoma. Up to 15% of patients with myasthenia gravis have thymomas, but more than this benefit from thymectomy. Conversely about 30% of patients with thymoma have myasthenia gravis.
(b) Germ cell tumours.
(c) Thymolipoma — rare. Usually asymptomatic. Occasionally radiolucent due to fat content.
(d) Thymic carcinoid. May secrete ectopic adrenocorticotropic hormone or parathormone. Latter may be part of multiple endocrine adenopathy syndrome. Locally invasive and often give rise to distant metastases.
(e) Lymphoma. Relatively commonly involved.
2 *Non-neoplastic.* Thymic cysts. Intrathymic haemorrhage.
*Calcification within thymic masses*:
(a) Coarse — in benign or malignant thymomas; germ cell tumours, especially teratomas.
(b) Peripheral/curvilinear — in thymic cysts; thymomas; cystic teratomas.

*Thymic hyperplasia* occurs in thymic 'rebound' after stress atrophy, and in a variety of endocrine and autoimmune states, e.g. thyrotoxicosis, Addison's disease, acromegaly, scleroderma, rheumatoid arthritis. The hyperplasia present in the majority of patients with myasthenia gravis is usually microscopic and not accompanied by macroscopic enlargement.

CT is the imaging method of choice after standard radiography. Up to one third of thymomas detected at CT are not visible on routine chest radiographs.
**REF: R214**

**A161** **a** *True* **b** *False* **c** *False* **d** *False* **e** *True*
*Fracture of a bronchus* is an uncommon injury but is usually

associated with trauma to other major mediastinal structures. Fractures of the upper three ribs are a common accompaniment of fractures of trachea or bronchi (>90%). These rib fractures, combined with a rapidly progressive pneumothorax, pneumomediastinum, or subcutaneous emphysema and a collapsed lung, strongly suggest tracheobronchial injury. The trachea usually fractures just above the carina. Bronchial fractures usually involve mainstem bronchi (80%), more common on the right. Pneumothorax occurs in 70%. In the rest the fracture is within the mediastinum with an intact medial parietal pleura. Mediastinal and subcutaneous emphysema are then seen. With complete bronchial transection and pneumothorax, the lung 'falls away' from the mediastinum to the most dependent aspect of the thorax.

Displacement of fracture margins may produce bronchial obstruction and collapse of the entire lung. In 10% no immediate radiographic abnormality is discernible since the bronchial sheath remains intact. Later, bronchial stenosis may occur with resulting atelectasis.

**REF: R215**

# Cardiovascular System

**A162  a** *True*  **b** *False*  **c** *True*  **d** *False*  **e** *True*

Some recognized associations

| | |
|---|---|
| *Down's syndrome* | Endocardial cushion defect, ventricular septal defect (VSD), atrial septal defect (ASD), Fallot's tetralogy, patent ductus arteriosus |
| *Turner's syndrome* | Coarctation of aorta, aortic stenosis |
| *Noonan's syndrome* | Pulmonary valvular stenosis |
| *Marfan's syndrome* | Aortic incompetence, mitral valve prolapse, aortic dissection |
| *Infantile hypercalcaemia* | Supravalvar aortic and pulmonary stenosis, peripheral pulmonary artery stenosis |
| *Congenital rubella* | Peripheral pulmonary artery/supravalvar stenosis, septal defects |
| *Secundum* ASD | Prolapsing mitral valve |
| *Primum* ASD | Cleft mitral valve + mitral regurgitation. +/− tricuspid regurgitation +/− heart block |
| *Sinus venosus* ASD | Partial anomalous pulmonary venous drainage |
| *Right-sided aortic arch* | In 30% of Fallot's<br>In 20% of transpositions<br>In 50% of truncus arteriosus<br>VSD<br>Vascular rings with anomalous left subclavian artery |
| *Holt-Oram syndrome* | See **A170** |
| *Maternal diabetes* | See **A167** |

**A163  a** *False*  **b** *True*  **c** *False*  **d** *True*  **e** *True*
*Thoracic aortic coarctation* is of two main types:
1 *Juxtaductal* ('adult type') — just distal to left subclavian origin.
2 *Diffuse hypoplastic* ('infantile type') — longer segment, often including left subclavian and common carotid. There is enough overlap in age of presentation for the 'adult' and 'infantile' labels to be discarded. There is a high incidence of patent ductus

arteriosus as well as cardiac defects, particularly those resulting in diminished flow through the aortic arch. Examples of these include bicuspid aortic valve and, less often, VSD and ASD.

*Presentation:*
(a) Symptoms within the first 2–3 months of life due to left ventricular failure.
(b) Later in life, usually related to investigation for hypertension.

*Chest radiograph:*
In infants there is cardiomegaly with pulmonary oedema indistinguishable from several other causes (see below). In the older group:
(a) Normal heart size, but left ventricular hypertrophy.
(b) 'Figure 3' appearance at aortic arch, usually due to dilated left subclavian and post stenotic dilation of aorta.
(c) Rib notching, usually not before 6 years old, only occasionally in infants. Unilateral-left sided notching is due to an anomalous right subclavian artery arising distal to the coarctation. Unilateral right-sided rib notching occurs when the left subclavian artery is involved in the coarctation.
(d) Dilated internal mammary arteries seen on the lateral view retrosternally.

*Complications:* Subacute bacterial endocarditis; aortic dissection; aortic sinus aneurysm; intracerebral berry aneurysms.
**REF: R216**

*Causes of heart failure in neonates/early infancy:*
(a) Hypoplastic left heart syndrome (most frequent).
(b) Massive left to right shunt (VSD with normal pulmonary vascular resistance).
(c) Obstructed total anomalous pulmonary venous return.
(d) Coarctation of aorta.
(e) Supravalvar aortic stenosis.

**A164**  a *True*  b *False*  c *True*  d *True*  e *True*

a Although *asplenia syndrome* (right isomerism; bilateral right handedness) and *polysplenia* syndrome (left isomerism; bilateral left-handedness) are described separately there is much overlap between them, some patients having features of both syndromes. Better terms may be 'visceroatrial situs ambiguous' with asplenia or polysplenia. Both syndromes have a high incidence of: total anomalous pulmonary venous drainage;

bilateral superior vena cava; ASD or common atrium; atrioventricular septal defect; VSD; transposition; cardiac malposition.
In asplenia there is a large bilaterally symmetrical liver, bilateral trilobed lungs, bilateral SVC's and IVC's, and, often cyanotic congenital heart disease with pulmonary stenosis. In polysplenia there is absence of the gall bladder, bilateral bilobed lungs, IVC interruption with continuation as the azygos vein; there may be acyanotic left-to-right shunt, total anomalous pulmonary venous drainage, or drainage of right pulmonary veins to right atrium and left pulmonary veins to left atrium (**REF: R217, R218**).
**b** Supravalvar, pulmonary trunk and peripheral pulmonary stenoses are associated with infantile hypercalcaemia and congenital rubella. There may be coexistent congenital heart disease.
**c** See **A162**.
**d** See **A166**.
**e** *Supravalvar aortic stenosis* may be familial, and may be associated with infantile hypercalcaemia. Pulmonary artery stenosis is often also present. It has also been reported in congenital rubella.

A165 **a** *False* **b** *True* **c** *True* **d** *True* **e** *False*
Eight defects account for about 90% of all congenital heart diseases: VSD (30%); ASD (10%); pulmonary stenosis (10%); patent ductus arteriosus (10%); Fallot's tetralogy (10%); aortic stenosis (7%); coarctation of aorta (5%); transposition (5%).

|  | Cyanotic | Non-cyanotic |
| --- | --- | --- |
| *Pulmonary plethora* | Transposition | ASD |
|  | Total anomalous pulmonary venous drainage | VSD |
|  | Truncus arteriosus | Aorto-pulmonary defect Patent ductus arteriosus |
| *Pulmonary oligaemia* | Tetralogy of Fallot Tricuspid atresia Pulmonary stenosis Ebstein's anomaly |  |

Note: all the 'T's are cyanotic!

*Some characteristic cardiac configurations*

| | |
|---|---|
| 'Snowman'/'figure of eight' | Total anomalous pulmonary venous drainage |
| Coer-en-sabot | Fallot's tetralogy |
| Narrow pedicle | Transposition of great vessels |
| Left sided ascending aorta + straight left heart border | Corrected transposition |
| Concavity in left heart border due to small pulmonary trunk + left atrial enlargement | Tricuspid atresia |

**A166**   a *False*   b *False*   c *False*   d *True*   e *True*

ASD is the most likely diagnosis in a non-cyanotic patient over the age of 3 years with pulmonary plethora. Clinical presentation can be at any age.

Radiological features on plain chest radiography in the uncomplicated case include:
1 Mild cardiomegaly.
2 Enlargement of right ventricle and right atrium.
3 The left atrium is normal or only slightly enlarged unless there is coexisting mitral prolapse or left ventricular dysfunction (cf. enlarged in VSD).
4 Left ventricle normal in uncomplicated ASD (cf. mostly normal in VSD).
5 The aortic arch is normal or small.
6 The central pulmonary arteries/pulmonary trunk are enlarged in the large majority (cf. mostly normal in VSD).
7 Peripheral pulmonary vessels are almost always plethoric. The degree will depend on the size of shunt and the pulmonary vascular resistance. Similar factors are important in VSD, but there may be normal pulmonary vasculature with small VSDs. High pulmonary vascular resistance may lead to the Eisenmenger syndrome of reversal of shunting. This is preceded by 'pruning' of the peripheral pulmonary arteries.
8 Calcification in central pulmonary arteries may occur in long-standing pulmonary arterial hypertension.
9 Dilatation of the superior vena cava at its lower end is sometimes seen in sinus venosus ASD with anomalous pulmonary venous drainage.
10 Associations of secundum ASD include: mitral valve prolapse +/− regurgitation; Lutembacher syndrome −

# Cardiovascular System 157

ASD + mitral stenosis; sinus venous type ASD is associated with partial anomalous pulmonary venous drainage.
Complications include Eisenmenger syndrome and bacterial endocarditis.
**REF: R219, R220**

**A167** a *True* b *False* c *True* d *False* e *True*
*Aortic sinus aneurysm* may be congenital, or acquired due to bacterial endocarditis. Incidence in the right and non-coronary sinuses is about equal: left sinus involvement is rare. Rupture produces a fistula from the right and non-coronary sinus aneurysms into the right atrium or right ventricle, i.e. a left-to-right shunt with a resulting variable degree of pulmonary plethora. The sinus is occasionally large enough to be seen on plain CXR; calcification is sometimes seen. Rupture of the rare left sided aneurysm is usually into the pericardial cavity with rapid death (**REF: R221**).

*Congenital pulmonary stenosis* may be valvar, supravalvar (see **A162** and **A164**), or infundibular (as in Fallot's tetralogy). Poststenotic dilatation is present in 90% of cases of valvar stenosis, but is unusual in the others. The pulmonary trunk in infundibular stenosis is usually normal or small (**REF: R221**).

*Atrial myxoma* occurs on the left in 75%. They are pedunculated intracavitary tumours, causing atrioventricular valve obstruction, often intermittent (causing a temporally variable degree of pulmonary oedema often with a normal sized left atrium), and occasionally accompanied by evidence of regurgitation. They present typically in the 30–60 age group. They are friable and give rise to emboli. Systemic symptoms are common, namely fever, weight loss, anaemia, clubbing and arthralgia. There is a raised erythrocyte sedimentation rate and serum gammaglobulins. Calcification in the tumour may be visible in 10%. Echocardiography will usually confirm the diagnosis (**REF: R221**).

*Carcinoid syndrome* frequently involves the heart. Usually the right side is involved, related to release of serotonin and related substances from liver metastases. However, the left side of the heart is occasionally affected. Tricuspid regurgitation and pulmonary valve stenosis are the commonest lesions. Tricuspid stenosis and pulmonary regurgitation are less frequent (**REF: R222**).

Infants of diabetic mothers have an incidence of congenital heart disease about four times that of controls. Commonest anomalies include VSD and abnormalities of the great vessels. In addition, two types of cardiomyopathy occur. A non-obstructive variety is due to poor left ventricular function and causes congestive heart failure. The obstructive form is indistinguishable from familial hypertrophic obstructive cardiomyopathy (HOCM) and is related to left ventricular outflow obstruction. Diagnosis is made by echocardiography. Unlike HOCM, the condition resolves in infancy (**REF: R131**).

A168  a *False*  b *True*  c *True*  d *False*  e *True*

*Patent ductus arteriosus*
The aortic knuckle is normal or enlarged (50%), providing a differentiating feature from intracardiac left-to-right shunts.

Premature infants are prone to delayed closure of the ductus. The normal degree of 'physiological pulmonary hypertension' that protects full-term infants from significant shunts is not as well developed in premature infants. Cardiac failure is therefore more likely to occur and to be more serious.

In premature infants with hyaline membrane disease enlargement of the heart, perhaps accompanied by increased shadowing in the lungs after initial improvement, often points to the development of pulmonary oedema secondary to a patent ductus. Ultrasonography can demonstrate the enlargement of the pulmonary artery, aorta, left ventricle and left atrium that accompany a patent ductus, but visualization of the ductus itself is difficult. However, Doppler examination is useful in detecting the turbulence in the pulmonary artery caused by the shunt. This may be aided by injection of agitated saline into an umbilical artery catheter which gives rise to microbubbles detectable as they cross from aorta into pulmonary artery. Calcification in the ductus occurs in long-standing cases, usually when pulmonary hypertension is present (Eisenmenger syndrome).
**REF: R223**

A169  a *False*  b *True*  c *False*  d *True*  e *False*

*Cardiomyopathy* is a disease of heart muscle of obscure aetiology. Therefore ischaemic, valvular and congenital heart disease, and cor pulmonale are excluded.

Classification

|  | Primary<br>(heart muscle alone affected) | Secondary<br>(part of generalized disease) |
|---|---|---|
| *Congestive* | Idiopathic<br>Post-infective<br>Peri-partum<br>Alcoholic | Haemochromatosis<br>Collagen disease<br>Sarcoidosis<br>Myxoedema<br>Amyloidosis<br>Beri-beri<br>Diabetes |
| *Hypertrophic* | HOCM | Friedrich's ataxia |
| *Restrictive* | Endocardial fibroelastosis<br>Endocardial fibrosis | Amyloidosis |

The chest radiograph typically shows an enlarged globular-shaped heart and evidence of left-sided heart failure. Similar appearances may be seen in pericardial effusion, except that pulmonary vascularity is normal. Ultrasonography will differentiate the two conditions.
**REF: R224**

A170 a *True* b *False* c *True* d *True* e *False*
The *Holt-Oram syndrome* comprises congenital cardiac defects — usually ASD, sometimes VSD — absent or finger-like thumbs, and other anomalies (e.g. carpal fusion or hypoplasia, os centrale) (**REF: R106**).

*Joint hypermobility* may be associated with mitral regurgitation in Marfan's syndrome and Ehlers-Danlos syndrome. The other features of Ehlers-Danlos include fragility of blood vessels, subcutaneous calcification, skull and spinal anomalies, cardio-vascular defects (aortic stenosis, aortic regurgitation, mitral regurgitation, aortic dissection, aneurysms, rupture of arteries), and spontaneous pneumothorax. Features of Marfan's syndrome include arachnodactyly, dolichocephaly, long limbs, lens dislocation,

kyphoscoliosis, atlanto-axial instability, cardiovascular defects (mitral valve prolapse/incompetence, aortic regurgitation, aortic enlargement and dissection) (see **A66**) (**REF: R106**).
Sarcoidosis, when it affects the heart, usually does so by causing cor pulmonale due to chronic lung disease. However, primary cardiac involvement does occur and is usually part of widespread sarcoid disease. Granulomas deposited in the heart cause conduction defects, including heart block, and cardiomyopathy. Rarely pericarditis or valve involvement may occur.

**A171**   **a** *False*   **b** *True*   **c** *True*   **d** *False*   **e** *False*
*Dressler's syndrome* (post-myocardial infarction syndrome) usually starts 1–6 weeks after infarction. Clinical and corresponding radiological manifestations include pleuritis with pleural effusion, pericarditis and pneumonitis. There is associated pleuropericardial pain, fever, arthralgia, raised peripheral white count, and raised erythrocyte sedimentation rate. ECG shows a pericarditis, apart from pre-existing ischaemic changes. The condition responds to salicylates, indomethacin or corticosteroids, but may recur. It is possibly related to an autoimmune mechanism, circulating antibodies to myocardium being present. A similar syndrome is described following cardiac surgery (post-pericardiotomy syndrome) and spontaneous trauma, leading to the adoption of the generic term 'post-cardiac injury syndrome'.

**A172**   **a** *True*   **b** *True*   **c** *False*   **d** *True*   **e** *False*
*Prolapsing mitral valve* ('floppy mitral valve') usually involves the posterior cusp which balloons into the left atrium in systole. Regurgitation is usually absent or slight. Five to ten per cent of the population have evidence of mitral valve prolapse on examination. The majority are asymptomatic healthy young females. Some patients have atypical chest pain and/or arrhythmias.
Associations:
1 Generalized connective tissue disorders — Marfan's syndrome; Ehlers-Danlos syndrome; osteogenesis imperfecta; relapsing polychondritis; lupus erythematosus; mucopolysaccharidosis.
2 Rheumatic carditis.
3 Atrial septal defect — secundum type.
4 'Straight-back syndrome' — loss of normal thoracic kyphosis

## Cardiovascular System 161

and reduction of the AP diameter of the thorax.
5   Pectus excavatum +/- straight back.
**REF: R225, R226**

A173   **a** *True*   **b** *True*   **c** *False*   **d** *False*   **e** *True*

*Central cyanosis* — decreased arterial oxygen tension. Affects mucous membranes and skin.
Causes:
1   *Impaired pulmonary function.*
(a) Alveolar hypoventilation (e.g. acute — pneumonia, pulmonary oedema. Chronic — chronic obstructive airways disease).
(b) Mismatched perfusion/ventilation.
(c) Diffusion block.
2   *Right-to-left shunts* (cyanotic congenital heart disease, including Fallot's tetralogy).
3   *Haemoglobin with low oxygen affinity.*
4   *Other haemoglobin abnormalities.*
(a) methaemoglobinaemia — hereditary and acquired.
(b) sulphaemoglobinaemia — acquired.
Cyanosis is apparent when the level of deoxygenated haemoglobin reaches 5 grams per 100 ml. Severe anaemia precludes central cyanosis since there is not enough reduced haemoglobin to produce cyanosis. Carboxyhaemoglobin, produced by carbon monoxide exposure, is incapable of carrying oxygen; carbon monoxide has a very high affinity for haemoglobin and displaces oxygen. A cherry-red colouration to skin and mucous membranes is seen.

A174   **a** *False*   **b** *False*   **c** *False*   **d** *True*   **e** *True*

*Radionuclide imaging of myocardium*
Thallium -$^{201}$ imaging detects ischaemic or infarcted myocardium by demonstrating it as a photopenic (i.e. 'cold') defect. Non-ischaemic, ischaemic (but viable), and infarcted muscle can be differentiated. A defect present at rest which takes up radionuclide on images obtained several hours later ('redistribution') indicates ischaemic but viable myocardium.
    Tc-labelled pyrophosphate myocardial scintigraphy is a sensitive indicator of acute myocardial infarction (>90% overall sensitivity), although the sensitivity is lower for subendocardial infarcts. However, other conditions lead to increased uptake in

the heart, although the uptake is usually more diffuse than in infarction. These include: previous myocardial infarction; angina; ventricular aneurysm; pericarditis; cardiomyopathy. Sensitivity in acute myocardial infarction for pyrophosphate scintigraphy peaks at 48–72 hours post-infarct, and gradually diminishes over the subsequent 2 weeks. Persistently positive imaging is an indicator of poorer prognosis.

Thallium-$^{201}$ scintigraphy shows acute myocardial infarction during the first few hours after infarction and turns negative after 1–2 days (**REF: R227, R228**).

A175 a *False*  b *True*  c *True*  d *False*  e *True*
*Pure mitral stenosis* is not a cause of left ventricular enlargement. However, associated significant regurgitation is.

*Tricuspid atresia* to be compatible with life, must be accompanied by septal defect. Blood then passes from right atrium to left atrium and left ventricle. The left ventricle maintains systemic and pulmonary circulations and is, therefore, enlarged.

An *anomalous left coronary artery* arises from the pulmonary trunk. Severe ischaemia of the left ventricle causes death in infancy, or patients may survive to present with early onset of ischaemic heart disease. Left ventricular enlargement is present due to heart failure or associated mitral regurgitation.

In *truncus arteriosus* with increased pulmonary blood flow there is enlargement of all four chambers of the heart. Both ventricles act as a common pumping chamber.

*Causes of left ventricular enlargement*:
1 Systemic hypertension.
2 Mitral regurgitation.
3 Aortic stenosis and regurgitation.
4 Ischaemic heart disease.
5 VSD.
6 Aorto-pulmonary shunts.
7 Cardiomyopathy.
8 Tricuspid atresia.
9 High output states, e.g. anaemia, peripheral arteriovenous shunts, thyrotoxicosis.

A176 a *True*  b *False*  c *False*  d *False*  e *False*
Signs of *pericardial effusion* on CXR include:
1 Large globular cardiac shadow, often increasing in size rapidly.

# Cardiovascular System 163

2 Changes in cardiac shape with posture.
3 Typically no pulmonary congestion or SVC dilatation.
4 Sharp outlines to the cardiac silhouette, due to diminished pulsation.
5 Enlargement of the cardiac shadow occurs predominantly anteriorly and laterally. Posterior enlargement is limited by the pulmonary veins.
6 Separation of epicardial and anterior mediastinal fat pad (**REF: R229**).
Echocardiography provides the best means of diagnosis.

*Differential diagnosis of massive cardiac enlargement*: pericardial effusion; mixed aortic and mitral valve disease; cardiomyopathy; Ebstein's anomaly.

*Causes of pericardial effusion*
1 *Inflammatory*.
(a) Infective. Viral (especially Coxsackie B); tuberculosis; rarely pyogenic.
(b) Non-infective. Rheumatic fever; radiotherapy; connective tissue disease (rheumatoid arthritis, systemic lupus erythmatosus); post-cardiac injury syndrome (e.g. Dressler's syndrome).
2 *Neoplastic*. Metastatic/direct spread — especially carcinoma of bronchus; lymphoma.
3 *Metabolic/endocrine*. Myxoedema; uraemia.
4 *Trauma*. Spontaneous — penetrating and blunt. Surgical.
5 *Severe congestive cardiac failure of any cause*.
**REF: R230**


A177  a *True*  b *True*  c *False*  d *True*  e *True*
Plain chest radiograph in *thoracic aortic dissection* may show:
1 Enlarged aorta or mediastinal widening (40–50%).
2 Loss of definition of aortic arch.
3 Tracheal deviation to the right.
4 Downward displacement of left main bronchus.
5 Displacement of intimal calcification >6 mm from the outer contour of aorta — the most specific sign.
6 Non-specific signs of mediastinal haemorrhage include: small left pleural effusion and the 'apical cap' sign.
Thoracic aortic dissections now tend to be classified as *proximal* (involving the ascending aorta whatever the extent) or *distal* (arising in or distal to the arch). The de Bakey classification is

now less used. This reflects the importance of the crucial question to be answered with regard to management — proximal dissections are treated surgically; distal dissections are usually treated conservatively, although some require surgery. CT is highly accurate in the diagnosis of dissection and also defines the type (proximal or distal). It is unable to assess blood flow in aortic branches (cf. aortography) but this is not of prime importance since management is based on clinical criteria. CT also cannot image the coronary vessels, and angiography may be required if a proximal dissection is demonstrated. Similarly aortic regurgitation is not visualized; arteriography is superior, but clinical examination and ultrasound are usually diagnostic.

Echocardiography is accurate in the diagnosis of proximal dissections with very few false negatives, but some false positives. A suitable diagnostic algorithm would be to perform ultrasonography as the initial imaging investigation. A positive for proximal dissection would result in angiography and then surgery. Negative ultrasonography leads to CT. Proximal dissection or equivocal appearances on CT leads to angiography. Distal dissection on CT would usually obviate the need for aortography and lead to continued medical therapy. Negative CT essentially excludes dissection.

Causes of aortic dissection include: hypertension; Marfan's syndrome and cystic medial necrosis; Ehlers-Danlos syndrome; pregnancy; coarctation; trauma; iatrogenic (catheterization); congenital aortic stenosis.

**REF: R231, R232**

**A178**  a *True*  b *True*  c *False*  d *False*  e *False*

There are a considerable number of causes of *renal microaneurysms*. However, most are very uncommon. The most important causes are:
1  *Polyarteritis nodosa* and variants such as *allergic granulomatosis* (Churg-Strauss syndrome).
2  *Drug abuse.*
3  *Bacterial endocarditis* (myocotic aneurysms).
4  *Malignant hypertension.*
5  *Tuberous sclerosis.*

The common pathway for formation of microaneurysms in the polyarteritis nodosa (PAN) spectrum of diseases, and in drug abuse, is a necrotizing angiitis which is probably due to damage from circulating immune complexes and complement activation. In many drug abusers and about half of patients with

PAN, the antigen involved seems to be one of the Hepatitis-B antigens. The clinical, angiographic and histological findings in necrotizing angiitis due to PAN and drug abuse may be indistinguishable. Endarteritis obliterans is also seen in the kidney in PAN.
**REF: R233, R234**

A179 **a** *False* **b** *True* **c** *False* **d** *False* **e** *True*
*Signs of mediastinal haematoma on CXR:*
1 Widening of superior mediastinum.
2 Loss of definition or abnormality of aortic contour.
3 Deviation of nasogastric tube to the right.
4 Deviation of trachea to the right.
5 Left main bronchus deviated inferiorly and medially.
6 Apical pleural cap of fluid.
7 Left haemothorax.
8 Widened right paratracheal stripe.
9 Widened left paratracheal stripe.
These signs have shown varying specificities in different series. Mediastinal haematoma is not synonymous with aortic laceration. The most helpful signs for mediastinal haemorrhage are **1, 2, 3, 6** and **8**. One series (**R235**) suggests that only **3** and **8** point to those who are more likely to have an abnormal aortogram, and that if these two signs are absent, then there is a 90% probability of an aortic rupture being absent. The vast majority of aortic lacerations occur at the isthmus (90% of those patients reaching hospital). A few occur just above the aortic valve.
   The majority of individuals sustaining a laceration of the aorta die before reaching hospital. In the initial survivors there is a cumulative mortality of 90% at four months without surgery. There should therefore be a low threshold of suspicion for investigation for this condition, and discovery of an aortic injury is an indication for surgery. Aortography is the investigation of choice, although there is preliminary evidence that CT may be useful (**REF: R235–R237**).

A180 **a** *False* **b** *False* **c** *False* **d** *True* **e** *False*
*Mycotic aneurysms* are related to lodging of a septic embolus in the artery or vasa vasorum, usually at a point of bifurcation, and are usually associated with bacterial endocarditis. Less commonly, bacteria may spread to the artery from an adjacent focus of infection.

There is a strong association with intravenous drug abuse. Mycotic aneurysms are infrequent, but commoner sites include the aorta, mesenteric vessels, hepatic and splenic arteries and intracerebral arteries. Renal artery involvement is very rare. A well-recognized, but rare, occurrence is catastrophic bleeding from a mycotic aneurysm into a tuberculous cavity.

There is a great risk of rupture of mycotic aneurysms (75%). Thrombosis, however, rarely occurs.

**REF: R238, R239**


**A181**   a *True*   b *False*   c *False*   d *False*   e *True*
Causes of *calcification in arteries* include:
1   *Atherosclerosis* (atheroma).
2   *Monckeberg's medial sclerosis*. Common, occurring with increasing age. Increased incidence in diabetes mellitus, hyperparathyroidism and renal osteo-dystrophy. Especially major vessels of the lower limbs. Artery narrowing is usually due to coexisting atheroma.
3   Homocystinuria.
4   Pseudoxanthoma elasticum.
5   Hypervitaminosis D.

# Central Nervous System and Skull

**A182** **a** *True* **b** *True* **c** *False* **d** *True* **e** *False*
Causes of *basal ganglia calcification*:
1  Idiopathic — commonest.
2  Idiopathic familial (Fahr's syndrome).
3  Parathyroid: hypo-; pseudohypo-; pseudopseudohypo-; hyper-parathyroidism.
4  Congenital infections. Toxoplasmosis (also paraventricular and cortical), cytomegalovirus and rubella (often more paraventricular).
5  Following encephalitis lethargica.
6  Following anoxia.
7  Carbon monoxide poisoning.
8  Following radiotherapy.
9  Tuberose sclerosis (most commonly paraventricular).
10  Cockayne's syndrome.
CT has shown calcification of the basal ganglia to be more common than previously thought in asymptomatic patients.
**REF: R240**

**A183** **a** *True* **b** *False* **c** *True* **d** *False* **e** *True*
An optic canal of diameter 7 mm or above on standard radiography should be considered abnormal. However, comparison with the opposite side is more reliable — a difference of >1 mm is significant.
Causes of *widening of the optic canal*:
1  Optic nerve glioma.
2  Neurofibromatosis — due either to glioma or hyperplasia of optic nerve. One-quarter of patients with optic nerve glioma have neurofibromatosis.
3  Retinoblastoma — extra-ocular extension.
4  Vascular anomalies. Ophthalmic artery aneurysm; arterio-venous malformation.
5  Inflammatory processes. Sarcoid; non-specific granuloma; orbital pseudotumour.
Many extrinsic lesions cause local defects in the margins of the optic canal, e.g. carcinoma of the ethmoid and sphenoid sinuses

(medial wall), granuloma of the sphenoid (medial), raised intracranial pressure (thinning superiorly), meningioma or glioma (superior), conditions enlarging the superior orbital fissure (lateral and inferior).
**REF: R241**

A184    a *False*   b *False*   c *False*   d *False*   e *True*
*Myotonic dystrophy* is associated with a small pituitary fossa, a thick vault (due to cerebral atrophy), and, sometimes, enlarged frontal sinuses.

*Craniopharyngioma* is usually primarily suprasellar, but may extend into the pituitary fossa. Primarily intrasellar lesions only occur in 10%. Typically there is erosion of the top of the dorsum sellae. Enlargement of the fossa is much less frequent. Calcification occurs in 40% overall (80–90% in children, 20% in adults). Rarely craniopharyngiomas occur in the nasopharynx.

Differential diagnosis of suprasellar masses: craniopharyngioma; meningioma (olfactory groove); optic chiasm glioma; 3rd ventricle glioma; suprasellar aneurysm; ballooned 3rd ventricle.

*Prolactinoma* (see **A196**).

*Cushing's syndrome.* The classification of pituitary tumours on the basis of chromophobe, acidophil and basophil cells has been largely discarded since there is overlap of clinical and biochemical features between different histological varieties. Most patients with Cushing's syndrome have adrenal hyperplasia secondary to pituitary adrenocorticotrophic hormone overproduction (Cushing's disease). In those having pituitary tumours (mostly basophil), the tumours are very small and do not lead to enlargement of the pituitary fossa. But note that after adrenalectomy the fossa may enlarge (Nelson's syndrome) (see also **A197** and **A198**).

*Raised intracranial pressure* — enlargement of the pituitary fossa may accompany the later stages of erosion, which starts as erosion of the lamina dura. This usually begins at the anterior aspect of the dorsum near the base. Enlargement occurs by extension of erosion inferiorly and posteriorly.
**REF: R240**

A185    a *True*   b *False*   c *False*   d *True*   e *False*
Some causes of *multiple Wormian bones*: osteogenesis imperfecta; cleidocranial dysostosis; hypophosphatasia; pycnodysostosis;

# Central Nervous System and Skull

congenital hypothyroidism; otopalatodigital syndrome; normal variant.

**A186**   a *True*   b *True*   c *True*   d *False*   e *False*

*Causes of calcification in the orbit*
1 *Globe.*
  (a) Lens — cataract.
  (b) Vitreous/choroid — degenerative changes following trauma or infection.
  (c) Retinoblastoma.
  (d) Retrolental fibroplasia.
  (e) Hyperparathyroidism.
2 *Retro-bulbar.*
  (a) Meningioma of optic nerve sheath.
  (b) Invasion by osteomas of the paranasal sinuses.
  (c) Other tumours — dermoids, neurofibroma, carcinoma of lacrimal gland.
  (d) Phleboliths.
   (i) Venous malformation. Congenital presenting in infancy or childhood. Most numerous of the causes of orbital varices. 25% associated with extraorbital venous anomalies, e.g. scalp venous malformations. Radiographic signs — orbital enlargement, phleboliths, prominent venous markings in the frontal bone. Venous anomalies outside the head and neck — Klippel – Trenaunay syndrome.
   (ii) Cavernous haemangioma. Much less common than venous malformations.
**REF: R241**

**A187**   a *True*   b *True*   c *False*   d *False*   e *True*
Most of the causes of generalized increased bone density cause changes in the skull, such as *pyknodysostosis, osteopetrosis, fluorosis* (see **A90**).
    *Craniometaphyseal dysplasia,* an inherited disorder, causes sclerosis of skull vault and base and facial bones, as well as flaring of metaphyses of the tubular bones. In addition, conditions such as *Paget's disease* and *fibrous dysplasia,* although localized or of patchy distribution in the body, frequently affect the skull, including the base. Long-term *phenytoin* (Dilantin) therapy causes generalized thickening and increased density of the skull, which also affects the base.

170              Answers and Notes

Meningioma adjacent to the skull base may cause *localized* hyperostosis. Chordoma is characteristically a destructive lesion (see **A61**).

**A188**  a *False*  b *True*  c *False*  d *True*  e *True*
The following lesions calcify with varying frequency:
1 Masses arising primarily in the parasellar region include: meningioma; optic chiasm glioma; aneurysms of Circle of Willis or intracavernous internal carotid artery.
2 Masses extending into parasellar region from pituitary fossa or temporal lobe or adjacent bone: craniopharyngiomas; pituitary adenomas; temporal lobe gliomas; chordomas.
3 Lesions without mass effect including atheroma of the internal carotid artery and basal meningeal calcification from previous *tuberculous* meningitis.
**REF: R240**

**A189**  a *True*  b *True*  c *False*  d *True*  e *False*
Lesions which may be of increased attenuation relative to normal brain on CT (excluding calcified lesions):
1 *Tumours*.

| | |
|---|---|
| Meningioma | : typically slightly increased attenuation +/- calcification. Oedema, but may be slight. +/- hyperostosis. |
| Metastasis | : increased, decreased or mixed attenuation + marked oedema. |
| Microglioma | : 2 patterns: (a) low density infiltrating lesion with little or no enhancement. (b) discrete increased density mass with marked enhancement + oedema. |
| Glioma | : wide spectrum. A few increased, most decreased or mixed attenuation with variable oedema. |
| Medullo-blastoma | : slightly increased density or isodense. Midline in the region of the inferior vermis. Metastasizes in CSF pathways. |
| Pinealoma | : (a) true pineal tumours (calcify). (b) germinomas. (c) teratomas (calcify). (d) occasional gliomas or metastases. |
| Craniopharyngioma | : usually mixed attenuation. +/- calcification. Typically solid and cystic components. |

Central Nervous System and Skull 171

    Chordoma : clivus extending into nasopharynx. Bone erosion. Partially calcified.
    Choroid plexus
    papilloma : most often at trigone of lateral ventricle.
    Occasionally acoustic
    neuroma : most isodense without IV contrast
2  *Colloid cyst*. Rounded hyperdense mass in the anterior part of the third ventricle, usually with hydrocephalus.
3  *Haematoma*. Peripheral low attenuation and oedema.
4  *Haemorrhagic infarct*. Areas of increased density within decreased attenuation.
5  *Large aneurysm/arteriovenous malformation*.
6  *Acute subdural haematoma*. Increased density for first 10 days.
7  *Extradural haematoma*.
**REF: R240**

A190  a *True*  b *True*  c *False*  d *True*  e *False*
**a**  The lack of signal from surrounding bone and of the resulting artefact (a problem in CT of the posterior fossa) makes magnetic resonance imaging (MRI) very accurate in the delineation of posterior fossa tumours, especially those adjacent to bone (e.g. acoustic neuromas). CT is superior to MRI in the detection of bone erosion (**REF: R242**).
**b**  Lesions of multiple sclerosis show as high signal intensity, periventricular lesions on MRI. This follows from the excellent ability of MRI to differentiate white and grey brain matter (**REF: R243, R244**).
**c**  MRI is insensitive to small volumes of calcification (cf. CT). This leads to difficulty in diagnosing small calcium-containing meningiomas (see below).
**d**  MRI is able to demonstrate the lateral margins of subdural haematomas unobscured by bone. There are no problems with isodense subdural haematomas, as sometimes occurs with CT (**REF: R245**).
**e**  CT can give a more specific diagnosis of meningioma because of its greater sensitivity for calcification and the frequent accompanying hyperostosis, (as well as the typically dense enhancement with intravenous contrast medium). On MRI the T1 and T2 of meningiomas are close to that of normal tissue (**REF: R243**).
**REVIEW REF: R246**

**A191** **a** *True* **b** *True* **c** *True* **d** *False* **e** *False*
The following typically show marked enhancement:
1 *Tumours.*
(a) Meningioma. Characteristic site (adjacent to skull vault, base, the tentorium or falx — most frequently parasagittal, olfactory groove, sphenoid ridge or tentorial). Slightly denser than brain on plain CT, some contain calcification. Hyperostosis. Variable, but usually only slight oedema **REF: R247**.
(b) Acoustic neuroma. Usually isodense on plain CT, but marked enhancement. Therefore contrast medium should always be given if plain scan negative or equivocal.
(c) Ependymoma. Most frequently occurs in lining of fourth ventricle in midline in children, occasionally in lateral ventricles in adults. (Also commonest intramedullary spinal tumour.) Calcification not infrequent — also may be seen on plain X-ray. Usually denser than brain on plain CT.
(d) Microglioma. Primary lymphoma of brain (see **A189**).
(e) Metastasis. Nearly always enhance. Sometimes ring enhancement. Marked oedema.
(f) Glioma. Variable enhancement. A wide spectrum of CT appearances. The tendency is for the more malignant ones (glioblastoma, malignant astrocytoma) to be of mixed attenuation and show enhancement. Homogeneous low attenuation and no enhancement implies a benign glioma. Some calcification is not uncommon, but large amounts often imply low malignancy. Peripheral oedema common, difficult to differentiate from infiltration (**REF: R248**).
(g) Pinealoma (see **A189**).
(h) Choroid plexus papilloma.
2 *Aneurysm* (unless thrombosed; if partly thrombosed may show ring enhancement).
3 *Arteriovenous malformation.*
4 *Acute cerebral infarct.* Occasionally marked enhancement, but not typical. Enhancement may occur as soon as 6 hours. The appearances of cerebral infarcts show a wide variation, but the following are the most common patterns:

Central Nervous System and Skull 173

|  | 1st week | 2nd week | 3rd week |
|---|---|---|---|
| Attenuation | iso/low | low | lower/cystic |
| Definition | ill | better | sharp |
| Mass effect | 25% | gradual reduction | |
| Enhancement | 50%* | 90% whole or part, may be peripheral | |

* There is some evidence that IV contrast is deleterious and should be reserved for cases in which the diagnosis is in doubt.

A192 a *True* b *False* c *True* d *False* e *False*
*Von Hippel-Landau syndrome* consists of multiple CNS and ocular haemangioblastomas, usually in the subpial region of the cerebellum. They often also involve the medulla and spinal cord. 5–20% of patients with haemangioblastomas have other features of this syndrome. Cysts occur within solid abdominal organs. Other associations are polycythaemia (up to 20% of those with cerebellar lesions), renal cell carcinoma (10–35%), and phaeochromocytoma (**REF: R249**).

*Sturge-Weber syndrome* is the association of a naevus of the face or scalp (ophthalmic dermatome of trigeminal nerve) with localized or hemi-atrophy of the cortex and capillary naevus of the meninges which gives rise to parallel bands of superficial (*not* paraventricular) calcification suggesting the shape of gyri (**REF: R250**).

*Treacher-Collins syndrome* (mandibulofacial dysostosis) consists of a variety of malformations of the mandible and/or maxilla, and external auditory canal and defects of the auricles. The underlying disorder is arrested development of the first branchial arch and groove (**REF: R106**).

A193 a *True* b *True* c *False* d *True* e *False*
*Horner's syndrome* comprises unilateral miosis, ptosis, enophthalmos and diminished sweating of the face.
*Causes:* lesions affecting the sympathetic pathways in the brainstem; sympathetic tract in the cervical or upper thoracic cord; T1 nerve root; sympathetic chain in the neck; stellate ganglion or cervical sympathetic plexus. For example: brainstem — vascular or demyelinating disease; Pancoast

tumour — affects sympathetic plexus; syringobulbia; primary neoplasm in the neck or cervical lymph node; metastases; trauma to neck; carotid aneurysm.

A194  a *False*  b *False*  c *True*  d *False*  e *True*

*Acoustic neuroma*
a  Plain radiography shows widening of the internal auditory meati in about 50% of cases. Plain tomography demonstrates bone erosion better than plain radiography.
b  Acoustic neuromas are typically isodense on plain CT (about 5% are hyperdense).
c  Most show marked enhancement with intravenous contrast medium. In view of this and b, contrast should always be given if the plain CT is negative or equivocal.
d  The lack of signal from surrounding bone on MRI, makes acoustic neuromas easy to see (see **A190**). However, CT will obviously show bone erosion to better effect.
e  CT air meatography or MRI is the only sure method of excluding a small or intracanalicular acoustic neuroma (**REF: R240, R251, R252**).

A195  a *False*  b *False*  c *True*  d *False*  e *True*

**Subarachnoid haemorrhage (SAH)**
Clinical clues to the localization of the source of bleeding include:
1  3rd nerve palsy — usually origin of posterior communicating artery.
2  Transient paresis of one or both lower limbs — anterior communicating aneurysm.
3  Hemiparesis — middle cerebral aneurysm.
4  Unilateral blindness — ophthalmic artery, anterior communicating.
5  Akinetic mutism or mood change — anterior communicating aneurysm.
6  Side of headache and preretinal haemorrhage may lateralize the aneurysm.

*Sites of aneurysms found at angiography after SAH*
Junction anterior cerebral/anterior communicating arteries  30%

## Central Nervous System and Skull

| | |
|---|---|
| Origin of posterior communicating artery | 25% |
| Middle cerebral artery | 21% |
| Terminal internal carotid artery | 13% |
| (half of these occur inside the cavernous sinus, therefore do not produce SAH) | |
| Basilar | 3% |
| No aneurysm found at angiography | 25% |
| Multiple aneurysms | 15–22% |

*The role of CT in SAH*

CT should be performed as soon as possible.
1  Confirms blood in the subarachnoid space and thus obviates the need for lumbar puncture.
2  It may give direct evidence of an aneurysm, but angiography is still required.
3  Demonstration of other causative lesions in patients thought clinically to have had SAH
4  Demonstration of associated intracerebral and intraventricular bleeding.
5  Demonstration of associated subdural haematoma (5%).
6  Demonstrates mild hydrocephalus (10% in first week, 20% during second week). Occasionally clinically significant communicating hydrocephalus.
7  Evidence that there is a high correlation between the extent and site of clot seen on CT and vasospasm on subsequent angiography.

Cerebral vasospasm is the major cause of delayed morbidity in SAH. It is seen maximally at 4–14 days post-ictus. The role of angiography is to confirm an aneurysm and to provide the anatomical details necessary for surgery. It is most often performed as soon as the patient is fully conscious.
**REF: R253, R254**

A196  a *True*  b *True*  c *False*  d *False*  e *False*

*Prolactinoma*
Amenorrhoea is the commonest presenting feature of pituitary prolactinomas, followed in frequency by galactorrhoea. Less common symptoms include, oligomenorrhoea, infertility with normal menses and hirsutism. Males present with impotence or hypogonadism. Large tumours often cause visual field defect.
There is no direct correlation between tumour size and

prolactin levels, but a serum prolactin of more than 500 mg/ml is usually associated with a macroadenoma, Nelson's syndrome, acromegaly, pituitary hyperplasia, oral contraception, phenothiazines, isoniazid and reserpine.

Normal variants, including asymmetry of the dorsum of floor of the fossa and apparent local cortical thinning are often mistaken as signs of an intrasellar mass. Only 25% of prolactinomas have abnormalities on plain tomography. Direct coronal imaging by CT, with dynamic scanning following intravenous contrast medium injection, is the current imaging method of choice when suspecting a prolactinoma. In a recent series, however, true positive examinations were slightly less frequent than false positives. Microadenomas typically show as focal or hypodense lesions. There may be a mass effect with convexity of the superior surface, abnormal gland height, inferior bone erosions or infundibular displacement. Large adenomas tend to be more homogenous and more likely to show intense heterogenic enhancement or ring enhancement.
**REF: R255**

# Endocrine System and Metabolism

**A197**  a *False*  b *False*  c *True*  d *False*  e *False*

**Cushing's syndrome**
*Clinical features* — Obesity; hypertension; hirsutism; amenorrhoea; striae; bruising; oedema; diabetes mellitus; erythrocytosis; hypokalaemic alkalosis.
1 *Endogenous causes.*
(a) Adrenal hyperplasia (80%) — secondary to pituitary ACTH production (most have pituitary adenoma) — Cushing's disease.
(b) Adrenal neoplasm (19%) — adenoma (most), occasionally carcinoma.
2 *Exogenous/iatrogenic.*

**A198**  a *True*  b *False*  c *False*  d *False*  e *True*

*Radiological features of Cushing's syndrome*
Osteoporosis (mainly axial); pathological fractures, especially wedging of vertebrae; exuberant callus with fractures; widened mediastinum (fat); fatty infiltration of the liver; cardiomegaly; pulmonary oedema; ischaemic bone necrosis, especially of femoral and humeral heads; delayed skeletal maturation. Most patients with Cushing's syndrome have a normal pituitary fossa on plain radiography, apart from osteoporosis of the dorsum sellae, since adrenal hyperplasia secondary to increased pituitary ACTH is usually related to pituitary-hypothalamic dysfunction or a pituitary microadenoma.

*Adrenal tumours*

|  | Pathology | Bilaterality | Usual size |
|---|---|---|---|
| Cushing's | Hyperplasia Neoplasm | Yes Atrophy of contralateral gland | Variable |
| Conn's | Adenoma 75% | Unilateral 90% | Small <3 cm |
| Non-functioning adenoma | Adenoma | No | Small |
| Phaeochromocytoma | 10% malignant | 10% | Usually 2–4 cm |

REF: R256, R257

A199  a *False*  b *False*  c *True*  d *False*  e *True*

The rule of 10% is a mnemonic for *phaeochromocytoma*:
  10% are malignant
  10% are extra-adrenal
  10% of extra-adrenal phaeochromocytomas are extra-abdominal
  10% are bilateral in adults

Biochemical diagnostic screening is by measurement of urinary vanillylmandelic acid or metanephrine. Glucagon may precipitate an acute hypertensive episode. Phaeochromocytoma may be part of the multiple endocrine adenopathy syndrome type II (see **A207**) and is then associated with hyperparathyroidism. It is also associated with the congenital neuroectodermal disorders (neurofibromatosis, tuberose sclerosis, von Hippel-Lindau syndrome).

A200  a *False*  b *True*  c *True*  d *False*  e *True*

*Causes of adrenal calcification*
1  *Prior haemorrhage*. Friderichsen-Waterhouse syndrome. Usually associated with septicaemia — often meningococcal. Rarely occurs in anticoagulant treatment, and as a complication of adrenal venography.
    The normal neonatal adrenals are large. Occasionally

haemorrhage occurs from traumatic breech delivery or perinatal sepsis. Calcifications form, and, after several months the glands have shrunk to a triangular calcified mass.
2 *Infection*. Tuberculosis; histoplasmosis.
3 *Associated with Addison's disease*. Previously were mostly due to tuberculosis. Now mainly auto-immune atrophy, associated with Hashimoto's thyroiditis and pernicious anaemia.
4 *Neoplasms*. Most common in malignant neoplasms. Up to 50% of neuroblastomas. Also frequent in ganglioneuromas. Rare on plain radiography in phaeochromocytoma — amorphous or egg-shell — but in about 7% on CT. Adrenal carcinomas are usually large at presentation and may contain irregular calcification. Calcification is extremely rare in Conn's tumours.
5 *Benign cyst* — may be part of post-haemorrhage spectrum (see above). Curvilinear calcification.
6 *Idiopathic*.
7 *Wolman's disease*. A rare congenital lipoidosis.
REF: R258


A201 a *True*  b *True*  c *False*  d *False*  e *False*
CT is the primary imaging modality of choice in disease of the adrenal cortex or medulla, and is often the only one required. It is highly accurate in the detection or exclusion of adrenal masses. False negatives occur in tumours <1 cm in size. CT is not reliable in the distinction of normal from hyperplastic glands (in Cushing's or Conn's syndrome), but it is the recognition of a tumour that is the only relevant distinction. Radionuclide imaging with I–131 labelled cholesterol derivatives is effective in Cushing's syndrome and primary hyperaldosteronism, but takes longer to perform, costs more, and involves a higher radiation dose. Selective adrenal vein sampling is the 'gold-standard' but is rarely required where CT and sophisticated biochemical tests are available.
    Ultrasound examination is not reliable, since the adrenals, especially the left, can be very difficult to visualize. However, when the adrenals are well seen and appear to be normal, the negative predictive value is high. In phaeochromocytoma, I-131-MIBG is better than CT at demonstrating extra-adrenal tumours and metastases of malignant phaeochromocytomas. It is useful for detecting multiple tumours, especially in patients with multiple endocrine neoplasia syndromes. Primary hyperaldosteronism is associated with a small, unilateral

cortical adenoma in >50% of patients, and bilateral hyperplasia in the rest. Bilateral tumours are rare. CT detects up to 75% of the adenomas, and should be the initial imaging test. If the CT is normal, then adrenal vein sampling and/or radionuclide imaging may be considered.

Labelled cholesterol derivatives are taken up by Conn's adenomas, which are thus seen as photon-abundant lesions. Most cases of Cushing's syndrome are due to overstimulation of the adrenals by the pituitary. Dexamethasone, an exogenous steroid, inhibits ACTH production, and thus cortisol levels, by negative feedback on the hypothalamic-pituitary axis in normals and in those with pituitary-derived Cushing's syndrome. Failure of suppression with high doses suggests an adrenal adenoma or ectopic ACTH production (see also **A197** and **A198**).
**REF: R257, R259**

A202  a *True*  b *True*  c *False*  d *True*  e *False*

*Grave's disease* is a condition of probable autoimmune aetiology, comprising hyperthyroidism, with diffuse toxic goitre, ophthalmic manifestations (lid-lag, lid-retraction, exophthalmos, ophthalmoplegia), and pretibial myxoedema. The latter feature may be accompanied by *thyroid acropachy*, and may occur during the active phase of thyrotoxicosis or after treatment. *Simple colloid goitre* may be endemic or sporadic, and results from the inability of the thyroid gland, in its basal state, to maintain the hormonal requirements of the body. This in turn may result from a variety of factors, such as iodine deficiency, congenital errors of metabolism, or following ablative thyroid treatment. Initially there is no associated thyrotoxicosis or myxoedema.

*Medullary carcinoma of the thyroid* demonstrates gross calcification within the primary tumour in about 10%. Similar calcification may be seen in metastases. There is often a desmoplastic reaction to the tumour caused by amyloid production. In *multiple endocrine neoplasia IIB (or III) syndrome* there is an association of phaeochromocytoma, medullary carcinoma of the thyroid and ganglioneuromatosis. The latter predominantly affects the face and mouth, but is also seen throughout the gastrointestinal tract. The colon is the most severely involved radiographically and may be striking. There are alternating regions of spasm and dilatation, and wall thickening. There may be a strong resemblance to congenital megacolon (see also **A207**).
**REF: R260**

## Endocrine System and Metabolism 181

**A203** a *False* b *False* c *True* d *False* e *True*

High resolution (10 MHz) real-time ultrasound, in the best hands, has a very high sensitivity for the detection of thyroid nodules. Although the typical appearance of thyroid carcinoma is of a poorly-defined mass which is hypoechoic relative to normal thyroid, and that of a benign adenoma is a large cystic component, a peripheral radiolucent halo, peripheral calcification and a hyperechoic texture, there is too much overlap to allow ultrasonography to make a reliable differentiation of benign from malignant nodules. Fine needle aspiration cytology is the most reliable non-surgical method of differentiating benign from malignant disease. A solitary nodule that is 'cold' on thyroid scintigraphy has a 15–25% chance of malignancy, whereas a 'cold' nodule in a multinodular gland has <1% chance of malignancy. Unfortunately, this situation probably cannot be extended to ultrasonography: in a patient with a clinically solitary thyroid nodule, the sonographic detection of a few additional nodules is probably not reliable for excluding malignancy, since the sensitivity for ultrasound detection of very small nodules is greater than for scintigraphy.
**REF: R261**

**A204** a *False* b *True* c *True* d *False* e *True*

In 85% of patients with *primary hyperparathyroidism* there is a solitary parathyroid adenoma.
The degree of hypercalcaemia in primary hyperparathyroidism is directly related to the size of the adenoma — in patients with severe hypercalcaemia the enlarged parathyroid is often palpable. Concomitant nodular thyroid disease exists in up to 40% of patients with primary hyperparathyroidism. There is also an increased incidence of thyroid carcinoma. Three non-invasive imaging modalities are available in the pre-operative localization of parathyroid adenomas:
1 High-resolution ultrasonography has an accuracy of up to 80% for localization and has an excellent specificity.
2 CT is reasonably good at demonstrating ectopic mediastinal adenomas. Variable results are achieved for adenomas in the normal position in the neck.
3 Double-tracer subtraction scintigraphy using $^{201}$-Tl-Thallous chloride (taken up by thyroid and parathyroids) and $^{99m}$-Tc pertechnetate (taken up by thyroid) is also

reasonably sensitive in parathyroid adenoma, and it is suggested that this technique and sonography are complementary tests.
REF: R262

**A205** a *False* b *True* c *False* d *True* e *False*

Some ectopic hormones produced by non-endocrine tumours

| Tumour osteomalacia | See **A83** |
|---|---|
| Serotonin (carcinoid) | Bronchial oat cell & adenoma |
| ACTH (Cushing's) | Bronchial oat cell (50%), bronchial carcinoid, islet cell tumour, thymus, medullary ca thyroid. |
| Inappropriate ADH | Oat cell and others of lung, pancreas, upper gastrointestinal ca. |
| Gynaecomastia | Choriocarcinoma, testis, bronchus. Squamous ca. bronchus, pancreas, ovary. |
| Pigmentation (melanocyte-stimulating hormone) | Oat cell bronchus. |
| Insulin-like | Retroperitoneal sarcoma Liver tumours (hepatoma). |
| Calcitonin | Medullary ca. of thyroid, breast, oat cell bronchus. |
| Erythropoetin | Cerebellar haemangioma, renal ca., liver tumours, uterus. |
| Hyperthyroid (thyroid secreting hormone) | Trophoblastic tumours choriocarcinoma, testis. |

REF: R79

**A206** a *True* b *True* c *False* d *True* e *True*
Physiological causes (self-limiting) — neonatal and adolescent.
  Pathological causes of *gynaecomastia* include:
  1 *Deficient male hormone*. Klinefelter's syndrome; testicular feminization; hypopituitarism; secondary testicular failure —

post-orchitis, trauma, castration, granulomatous disease, renal failure; congenital anorchia.
**2** *Increased oestrogen production.* Testicular tumours; carcinoma of bronchus; prolactinomas; adrenal tumours; cirrhosis; thyrotoxicosis; congenital adrenogenital hyperplasia; true hermaphroditism.
**3** *Drugs* — many but include: oestrogens; spironolactone; digoxin; cimetidine; narcotic abuse; tricyclic antidepressants; methyldopa.
**REF: R79**

**A207  a** *True*  **b** *True*  **c** *True*  **d** *True*  **e** *False*
The *Multiple Endocrine Neoplasia (MEN) syndromes* are familial conditions in which there is neoplasia (benign or malignant) and/or hyperplasia of multiple endocrine glands. Classification:
**1** *Type I.* The 'p's' — parathyroid, islet cell of pancreas, pituitary.
The islet cell tumour most frequently seen is a gastrinoma (Zollinger-Ellison syndrome). The resulting hypergastrinaemia is associated with intractable multiple peptic ulceration, often in unusual sites (such as distal duodenum, jejunum). In addition the hypercalcaemia caused by the parathyroid abnormality in these patients increases the propensity to ulceration, since it, too, causes hypergastrinaemia. Less commonly in MEN type I, the pancreatic tumour produces predominantly insulin. Abnormalities may also occur in thyroid and adrenal cortex. Occasionally carcinoid tumours occur **(REF: R263, R264)**.
**2** *Type IIA.* Medullary carcinoma of thyroid, phaeochromocytoma, parathyroid adenoma. Medullary carcinoma of the thyroid is derived from pluripotential C cells. There is a wide spectrum of aggressiveness. Primary tumour and secondary deposits tend to produce a marked desmoplastic reaction. A wide variety of substances is produced by the tumour including calcitonin, histaminase, amyloid, serotonin, bradykinin, ACTH. Consequently a variety of clinical symptoms occur. Diarrhoea occurs in 30%, with a rapid transit of barium. The phaeochromocytomas in the MEN syndrome are multiple in 50% (see **A199**).
**3** *Type IIB (or III).* Medullary carcinoma of thyroid, phaeochromocytoma, orofacial neuromas, characteristic facies.
The ganglioneuromas also affect the GI tract — see **A. 202**.
**REF: R260**

The *Verner-Morrison syndrome* (WDHA syndrome — Watery Diarrhoea, Hypokalaemia, Achlorhydria) is caused by a pancreatic apudoma that secretes Vasoactive Inhibitory Polypeptide -VIPOMA. This is usually sporadic, but a few cases are associated with MEN syndrome. (See **A.9**)
REF: R264

**A208**  a *True*   b *True*   c *False*   d *False*   e *True*

*Causes of hypokalaemia*
1  *Gastrointestinal loss.* Vomiting +/− diarrhoea; fistulas; villous adenomas; ureterosigmoidostomy.
2  *Poor dietary intake.*
3  *Renal loss.* Most diuretics (not spironolactone); osmotic diuresis (glycosuria); aldosteronism — primary (Conn's syndrome) and secondary to, for instance, malignant hypertension, liver disease; excess corticosteroids — Cushing's syndrome, steroid therapy, ectopic ACTH; renal tubular acidosis.
4  *Shift of potassium into cells.* e.g. insulin effect. Tubular necrosis and other causes of acute renal failure are usually associated with oliguria and hyperkalaemia. Addison's disease causes renal sodium loss and hyperkalaemia. Hypokalaemia is a cause of intestinal pseudo-obstruction (see **A26**).

**A209**  a *True*   b *True*   c *False*   d *False*   e *True*

*Radiological features of acromegaly*
1  *Overgrowth of soft tissues.* E.g. increased heel pad (see **A95**), spade-like digits, prominent entheses, carpal tunnel syndrome.
2  *Skull.* Thickened skull vault, frontal bossing, enlarged sinuses, enlarged pituitary fossa, prominent mandible.
3  *Axial skeleton.* Kyphoscoliosis, appositional bone growth to vertebral bodies leading to increased dimensions, posterior scalloping of vertebral bodies, enlargement of AP diameter of thorax, generalized osteoporosis.
4  *Peripheral skeleton.* Long bones thickened, 'spade-like' terminal tufts to digits, enlarged medial sesamoid index, generalized osteoporosis.
5  *Joints.* Widened joint spaces due to cartilage overgrowth, premature osteoarthrosis (but with relative preservation of joint space), chondrocalcinosis.
6  *Cardiomegaly.* Cardiomyopathy is a complication.

Endocrine System and Metabolism 185

Hypertension is a frequent accompaniment of acromegaly. Diabetes mellitus occurs in about 50%.
**REF: R88**

**A210**  a *False*  b *True*  c *False*  d *True*  e *True*
*Diabetes* is associated with calcified vasa deferens and seminal vesicles. Other causes of this include bilharzia and tuberculosis (rarely).
  Causes of *arthritis mutilans*: neuropathic joint disease including diabetes mellitus; rheumatoid arthritis; psoriatic arthropathy; juvenile chronic arthropathy; leprosy and chronic infection.
  Diabetes causes generalized retardation of bone maturation in childhood diabetics.
  Gastric ileus (acute gastric dilatation) is a reversible feature of diabetic ketosis. Delayed gastric emptying is a permanent manifestation of diabetic autonomic neuropathy.
  Diabetes is the predominant cause of bilateral renal enlargement (pathogenesis unknown). The preponderance of diabetes mellitus when this radiological finding is demonstrated is sufficient to recommend that fasting blood sugar estimation is performed in patients with unexplained bilateral renal enlargement (**R265**). Other causes of bilaterally enlarged smooth kidneys include: bilateral hydronephrosis; acute glomerulonephritis/vasculitis; infiltration with amyloid, myeloma, lymphoma, leukaemia; medullary sponge kidneys; acromegaly; polycystic disease (sometimes); acute tubular necrosis.

**A211**  a *False*  b *True*  c *False*  d *True*  e *True*
Major causes of *hypoglycaemia* include:
1 *Postprandial*. Previous gastric surgery (gastrectomy, gastroenterostomy, vagotomy) (see **A11**).
2 *Fasting*.
 (a) Underproduction of glucose
  Hormone deficiency:   hypopituitarism; adrenal insufficiency
  Enzyme defects:   glycogen storage disease
  Acquired liver disease:   cirrhosis; liver failure
  Drugs:   especially alcohol
 (b) Overutilization of glucose
  Hyperinsulinaemia:   insulinoma; exogenous insulin; sulphonylureas

Extrapancreatic
tumours:*                (retroperitoneal) fibromas and sarcomas; hepatoma; adrenal carcinoma; carcinoma of gastrointestinal tract

* Mechanism unknown — possibly due to substance with insulin-like activity.
**REF: R79**

# Miscellaneous Topics

**A212** **a** *False* **b** *True* **c** *False* **d** *True* **e** *False*
Signs of *splenic trauma* on plain abdominal radiography:
1 Left lower rib fracture: 45%.
2 Anteromedial displacement of the stomach.
3 Inferior displacement of the left kidney and left transverse colon.
4 Posterior extraperitoneal fat line: preserved with subcapsular haemorrhage; lost with intraperitoneal haemorrhage.
5 Mass in splenic fossa.
6 Injury to the left hemidiaphragm: 2%.
7 Signs of intraperitoneal blood: in pelvic recesses; in left paracolic gutter.

CT is a very accurate and simple method for detecting splenic injury. Intraparenchymal and subcapsular haematoma, lacerations, and intraperitoneal blood may be demonstrated (**REF: R266**). Although ultrasound may be valuable in splenic trauma (demonstrating enlargement, changes in contour, perisplenic fluid collection, subcapsular haematoma, parenchymal haematoma) examination is often limited due to local pain from accompanying rib fractures. Scintigraphy using Tc-labelled sulphur colloid is accurate in the diagnosis of splenic injury and is probably superior to ultrasound.

Abnormalities demonstrated on scintigraphy include a peripheral filling defect, a linear defect transecting or nearly transecting the spleen, fragmentation, or displacement.

Rarely avulsion of the spleen causes an absence of isotope uptake. Scintigraphy has also been employed to monitor progress in non-operative management of splenic trauma (**REF: R267**).

There is a trend towards conservative management of splenic trauma, especially in young patients, unless bleeding is uncontrolled, since splenectomy is associated with an increase in the incidence of septicaemia. The risk of delayed intraperitoneal rupture of a subcapsular haematoma is small.

**A213** **a** *False* **b** *True* **c** *True* **d** *False* **e** *True*
Causes of *calcification in the pinna* include: Addison's disease;

acromegaly; collagen diseases, e.g. scleroderma; relapsing polychondritis; gout; frostbite; ochronosis; trauma; chronic hypercalcaemia.
**REF: R88**

A214 **a** *True* **b** *True* **c** *False* **d** *False* **e** *False*
*Juvenile angiofibromas* are the commonest benign tumours of the nasopharynx. They most frequently occur between 7 and 21 years of age and are very rare in females. Presentation is with epistaxis and nasal obstruction. Arising in the area of the posterior nares, the tumour spreads assymetrically to both sides of the midline, through the pterygomaxillary fossa and may involve the paranasal sinuses, orbits, infratemporal fossa and cranium. Plain radiographic findings include: soft tissue mass in the nasopharynx; erosion of the floor of the sphenoid sinus, hard palate, pterygoid processes, medial wall of the maxillary antrum, floor of the orbit or superior orbital fissure; anterior bowing of the posterior antral wall — not absolutely specific but highly characteristic.
The tumours are highly vascular, and are supplied by branches of the external carotid artery. However, there are sometimes anastomoses between external and internal carotid artery branches — this may lead to complications when embolization of these tumours is attempted. CT, in keeping with the vascularity, demonstrates enhancement with intravenous contrast medium — the only extracranial tumour in this region that shows differential enhancement.
**REF: R268, R269**

A215 **a** *False* **b** *True* **c** *False* **d** *True* **e** *True*
Aortic coarctation is associated with intracranial berry aneurysms; patent ductus arteriosus is not.
*Klippel-Feil syndrome* consists of a short neck and low occipital hairline associated with fused cervical or cervico-thoracic vertebrae or other vertebral anomalies. Other associated abnormalities include atlanto-axial fusion, Sprengel shoulder, omovertebral bone. 30% are deaf due to various ear anomalies, e.g. absent auditory canal, deformed ossicles, hypoplastic bony labyrinth. The vertebral anomalies, or secondary spondylosis at adjacent levels, may lead to spinal block (**REF: R106**).
*Down's syndrome* is associated with various gastrointestinal tract anomalies including: duodenal atresia/stenosis, anorectal

# Miscellaneous 189

anomalies, Hirschsprung's disease, umbilical hernia.
*Neurenteric cysts* are duplication cysts associated with spinal anomalies. They may occur in the thorax or abdomen and are due to persistence of the embryological connection between primitive gut and neural tube. They may be open at one or both ends and communicate with the alimentary tract and/or the subarachnoid space (hence a thoracic meningocele). However, in most cases the connection is a fibrous cord without a lumen. Cysts may be lined with gastrointestinal epithelium. In particular they may present with bleeding due to acid production and ulceration. Various vertebral anomalies are associated including hemivertebrae and malsegmentation.

A216 a *True* b *True* c *True* d *False* e *True*
Complications of *narcotic drug abuse* affect multiple systems (see below). Increasingly, they may be part of the Acquired Immune Deficiency Syndrome (AIDS) which makes the addict susceptible to opportunistic infections.
Complications include:
1 *Pulmonary*.
(a) Reaction to the drug (e.g. pulmonary oedema).
(b) Infective — septic emboli, increased susceptiblity to 'ordinary' pneumonia, opportunistic infection (especially pneumocystis carinii — as part of AIDS).
(c) Kaposi's sarcoma — also part of AIDS. Most frequently involves skin, gastrointestinal tract, lymph nodes. Often associated with pneumocystis.
(d) Foreign body granulomas — talc granulomas. Contaminants of street drugs. Causes micronodulation which may progress to interstitial fibrosis (often predominantly upper lobe) and thence pulmonary hypertension.
2 *Musculoskeletal*.
(a) Soft tissues — mainly infective (local to site of injection or distant) and thrombophlebitis, and their consequences.
(b) Myonecrosis — local, causing muscle compartment syndrome; generalized, causing 'crush' syndrome of shock and renal failure.
(c) Bone and joints — infective complications, local or distant. Gram-negative organisms most common (cf. non-addicts). Non-tuberculous infective spondylitis is commonest site. Sternoclavicular and sacroiliac joints also relatively common. Incidence of tuberculous infection also increased.

3 *Vascular.* Thrombophlebitis; arterial occlusion; mycotic aneurysm; arteriovenous fistula; necrotizing angiitis — may be indistinguishable from polyarteritis nodosa, often associated with Hepatitis B antigen, affects the kidneys and gastrointestinal tract predominantly (see **A178**).
4 *Cardiac.* Bacterial endocarditis.
5 *Gastrointestinal.* Colonic pseudo-obstruction (see **A26**). Foreign bodies (concealment of drugs) — complications due to mechanical effects or leakage of drugs. Hepatitis — predominantly viral. Liver/spleen abscess. Necrotizing angiitis — see above. Necrotizing enteritis.
6 *Urinary tract.* Renal problems due to immune complex deposition, e.g. (a) nephrotic syndrome or membranous nephropathy associated with Hepatitis B antigen; (b) focal or diffuse glomerulonephritis associated with bacterial endocarditis; (c) heroin nephropathy — nephrotic syndrome due to focal glomerulosclerosis; (d) necrotizing angiitis. Renal amyloidosis also occurs. Renal abscess, fungal infections.
7 *Brain.* Multiple complications include consequences of trauma; ischaemic lesions related to episodes of hypoxia; opportunistic infections (AIDS); embolic phenomena due to endocarditis; mycotic aneurysm +/- SAH; atrophy.
**REF: R270-R275**

**A217** a *True* b *False* c *True* d *False* e *True*
Although it is very often impossible to distinguish *allergic* (vasomotor) from *infective sinusitis* on radiological grounds, and the two may frequently co-exist, the following features are typical of either entity:

|  | Allergic | Infective |
| --- | --- | --- |
| Distribution | Usually bilateral Commonly all sinuses | Often unilateral One or few sinuses |
| Thickened mucosa | Scalloped outline | Smooth, parallel to wall of sinus |
| Fluid levels | Rare | Common in acute phase |
| Nasal turbinates | Usually swollen | May be normal |
| Polyps | Common | Rare, but often retention cysts |
| Bone changes (chronic) | Decreased density in walls | Sclerosis of walls |

Mucous cysts are lined with epithelium and result from duct obstruction after infection. They are commoner than polyps and appear dome-shaped, broad-based and well-defined, often in the floor of the maxillary sinus and associated with thickened mucosa. Unlike polyps they do not move or change shape with changes in the position of the patient.
**REF: R268**

A218 a *True* b *True* c *False* d *False* e *True*
Causes of *scoliosis* include:
1 *Congenital*.
(a) Various vertebral anomalies including hemivertebra, failure of segmentation, supernumerary vertebrae. Progressive increase in curvature common. Congenital syndromes: neurofibromatosis; Marfan's syndrome; homocystinuria; VATER association; association with congenital heart disease; pulmonary hypoplasia.
2 *Idiopathic*.
(a) Infantile — recovers in >90%. Probably related to fetal malposition. Association with head moulding. A small number are progressive and severe.
(b) Juvenile and adolescent — progressive until vertebral growth ceases. Due to development of wedge-like deformity of the vertebral body and rotational defects.
3 *Neuromuscular disease*. Various muscular dystrophies; cerebral palsy; poliomyelitis; myelomeningocele.
4 *Postural*. E.g. leg length discrepancy.
5 *Acquired spinal disease*.
(a) Tumour — e.g. osteoid osteoma, osteoblastoma, neurofibroma. Myeloma or metastasis causing vertebral collapse.
(b) Infection.
(c) Degenerative — severe disc disease.
(d) Trauma.
(e) Following radiotherapy in childhood, e.g. for Wilm's tumour.
(f) Metabolic bone disease, e.g. osteoporosis.
6 *Muscular spasm*. E.g. renal colic, psoas abscess, acute appendicitis, perforated ulcer, subhepatic abscess. The spinal curvature is concave to the affected side.
**REF: R276**

**A219** a *True*  b *True*  c *False*  d *True*  e *False*

**Smooth masses in the breast**

Cysts and fibroadenomas are the commonest causes.

|  | Cysts | Fibroadenomas |
|---|---|---|
| Age | 30+, more often 40+ Rare under 30 years | Any age but especially under 30 |
| Association with pregnancy | Nil | 'Lactating' |
| Multiplicity | Often multiple | Single or multiple |
| Bilaterality | Common, often symmetrical situation | Sometimes, not symmetrical |
| Border | Typically well defined but may be obscured by surrounding breast tissue | Majority sharply circumscribed, may be obscured by surrounding breast tissue |
| Shape | Round or oval | Round or lobular |
| Sequential changes | May vary in size and number over a few months | May involute in older women. Occasionally grow after menopause. Tend to grow rapidly in teens and pregnancy |
| Calcification | Occasional peripheral curvilinear | Typically coarse 'popcorn' esp. in peri- and post menopausal women. May be fine and punctate in early stages |
| Association with carcinoma | Carcinoma rarely arises in wall of cyst | Very occasionally, small carcinoma found in close association |
| Ultrasound | Smooth margins, echo free interior, well defined posterior wall, enhanced transmission distally | Smooth contour, uniform weak internal echoes, well defined anterior and posterior margins |
| Aspiration | Clear fluid. Blood-stained may indicate rare associated carcinoma | Dry or blood |

## Miscellaneous

*Haematoma*
History of recent trauma (including biopsy) *but* trauma may lead to discovery of pre-existing carcinoma. Occasionally blood dyscrasia.
Mammography of haematoma: (a) ill defined mass with oedema and associated skin thickening or (b) well defined mass. Usually regresses and disappears in several weeks leaving no trace, but occasionally residual scarring or distortion. Calcifications may occur and are identical to those of fat necrosis (see below).

*Fat necrosis*
Also occurs after trauma or biopsy.
**1** *Mammography*. Typically a rounded, sharply circumscribed thin capsule surrounding an area of radiolucency (due to lipid material). Sometimes peripheral curvilinear calcification. Occasionally an ill defined mass, even containing irregular microcalcification which is indistinguishable from a carcinoma.
**2** *Galactocele* is another form of retained lipid material; mammographically seen as 1–1.5 cm round or oval areas of radiolucency, usually multiple and bilateral, sometimes with eggshell calcification.

*Other causes of a round, well defined breast mass*
**1** *Skin and subcutaneous masses* — e.g. naevi, moles, neurofibromata, sebaceous cysts.
**2** *Carcinoma*.
(a) **Medullary** (3% of all breast cancers).
(b) **Intracystic** — slight flattening of one border of a well defined rounded mass is suspicious of this rare type of cancer.
(c) **Intraductal, colloid and mucoid** producing cancers can also present as very well circumscribed masses, but often some irregularity or 'comet tail'.
**3** *Papilloma*. Most papillomas are invisible as they tend to be small and are within ducts. Occasionally are large, when subareolar in situation.
**4** *Intramammary lymph nodes*. Occur anywhere in breast, but usually upper/outer quadrants and axillary tail. Often multiple, usually bilateral. Usually less than 1 cm. Fat may be seen at hilus.
**5** *Cystosarcoma phylloides*. A fibroepithelial tumour that is benign or malignant. May mimic fibroadenoma. Often large, with well defined and lobulated margin. Occasionally contain very coarse calcifications.

6 *Lymphoma*. Primary in breast or part of diffuse disease. May be ill defined infiltrate or well defined ovoid or round mass.
7 *Metastases*. Apart from lymphoma and leukaemia, melanoma is the commonest metastasis to breast.
**REF: R277**

A220  a *True*  b *True*  c *False*  d *False*  e *False*

*Microcalcification*
Microcalcification is a product of increased cellular activity in the lobulo-ductal complex of the breast. Visible in 50% of carcinomas on xeroradiography and may be the only mammographic sign of cancer, in which case many of the tumours are *in situ* cancers. However, micro-calcification is seen in many forms of benign disease, e.g. sclerosing adenosis, intraductal hyperplasia, papillomatosis and fat necrosis. In general, large numbers of small calcifications in close aggregation, with non-rounded forms, increase the index of suspicion for carcinoma — although there are overlaps in the degree of these features with benign and malignant lesions. Linear, irregularly shaped or branching forms are especially likely to denote a carcinoma.
**REF: R277**

# References

R1  Donner M., Saba G.P. & Martinez C.R. 1981. Diffuse diseases of the esophagus: a practical approach. *Semin. Roentgenol.* **16**, 198–213.
R2  Ekberg O. 1981. Cervical oesophageal webs in patients with dysphagia. *Clin. Radiol.* **32**, 633–41.
R3  Bleshman M. *et al.* 1978. The inflammatory esophagogastric polyp and fold. *Radiology* **128**, 589–93.
R4  Williams S. *et al.* 1983. Work in progress: Tranverse striations of the esophagus: association with gastro-esophageal reflux. *Radiology* **146**, 25–7.
R5  McDermott P. *et al.* 1982. Double contrast examination of the oesophagus: the radiological changes in peptic oesophagitis. *Clin. Radiol.* **33**, 259–64.
R6  Bozymski E.M. *et al.* 1982. Barrett's oesophagus. *Ann. Intern. Med.* **97**, 103.
R7  Levine M.S. *et al.* 1983. Barrett esophagus: reticular pattern of the mucosa. *Radiology* **147**, 663.
R8  Goldstein H., Zornoza J. & Hopens T. 1981. Intrinsic diseases of the adult esophagus: Benign and malignant tumors. *Semin. Roentgenol.* **16**, 183–97.
R9  Moss A.A. 1982. Computed tomography in the staging of gastrointestinal carcinoma. *Radiol. Clin. North Am.* **20**, 761–80.
R10 Picus D. *et al.* 1983. Computed tomography in the staging of esophageal carcinoma. *Radiology* **146**, 433–8.
R11 Bruhlmann W. *et al.* 1981. Intramural pseudodiverticulosis of the esophagus: Report of 7 cases and literature review. *Gastrointest. Radiol.* **6**, 199–208.
R12 Ott D. *et al.* 1984. Esophagastric region and its rings. *Am. J. Roentgenol.* **132**, 281–7.
R13 Colin-Jones D. 1983. In: *Topics in Gastroenterology*: **12**. Ed. Jewell D.P. & Shepherd H.A. Blackwell Scientific Publications, Oxford.
R14 Laufer I. 1979. *Double Contrast Gastrointestinal Radiology with Endoscopic Correlation*. W.B. Saunders, Philadelphia.
R15 Feczko P. *et al.* 1985. Gastric polyps: Radiological evaluation and clinical significance. *Radiology* **155**, 581–4.
R16 Bouchier I.A., Allan R.N., Hodgson H.J. & Keighley M.R. 1984. *Textbook of Gastroenterology*. Bailliere Tindall, London.
R17 Koelz H. & Gewertz B. 1979. In: Post-surgical syndromes. *Clin. Gastroenterol.* **8**, 305–21.
R18 Alexander-Williams J. & Hoare A. 1979. In: Post-Surgical Syndromes. *Clin. Gastroenterol.* **8**, 321–53.
R19 Pilling D. 1983. Infantile hypertrophic pyloric stenosis: a fresh approach to the diagnosis. *Clin. Radiol.* **34**, 51–3.

R20  Meyers M. 1982. *Dynamic Radiology of the Abdomen.* 2nd Edition. Springer-Verlag, New York.
R21  Nolan D. & Gourtsoyiannis N. 1980. Crohn's disease of the small intestine: a review of the radiological appearances of 100 consecutive patients examined by a barium infusion technique. *Clin. Radiol.* **31**, 597–603.
R22  Jeffree M. *et al.* Primary carcinoid tumours of the ileum: the radiological appearances. *Clin. Radiol.* **35**, 451–5.
R23  Mendelson R. & Nolan D. 1985. The radiological features of chronic radiation enteritis. *Clin. Radiol.* **36**, 141–8.
R24  Bambach C. *et al.* 1981. Effect of intestinal surgery on the risk of urinary stone formation. *Gut* **22**, 257–63.
R25  Brunton F. & Guyer P. 1983. Malignant histiocytosis and ulcerative jejunitis of the small intestine. *Clin. Radiol.* **34**, 291.
R26  Bulow S. 1984. Colorectal polyposis syndromes. *Scand. J. Gastroenterol.* **19**, 289–93.
R27  Gardiner R. & Stevenson G. 1982. The colitides. *Radiol. Clin. North Am.* **20**, 797–817.
R28  Fishman M. *et al.* 1984. The dissection sign in nonreducible ileocolic intussusception. *Am. J. Roentgenol.* **143**, 5–8.
R29  Holt S. & Samuel E. 1978. Multiple concentric ring sign in the ultrasonographic diagnosis of intussusception. *Gastrointest. Radiol.* **3**, 307–9.
R30  Humphry A. *et al.* 1981. Perforation of the intussuscepted colon. *Am. J. Roentgenol.* **137**, 1135–8.
R31  Kogutt M. 1979. Necrotizing enterocolitis of infancy: early roentgen patterns as a guide to prompt diagnosis. *Radiology* **130**, 367.
R32  Warren G. & Kern F. 1983. The biliary tract in inflammatory bowel disease. *Clin. Gastroenterol.* **12**, 255–68.
R33  Allan R. 1983. Extra-intestinal manifestations of inflammatory bowel disease. *Clin. Gastroenterol.* **12**, 617–32.
R34  Loughran C., Tappin J. & Whitehouse G. 1982. The plain abdominal radiograph in pseudomembranous colitis due to Clostridium difficile. *Clin. Radiol.* **33**, 277–81.
R35  Kim S. *et al.* 1976. Cathartic colitis. *Am. J. Roentgenol.* **131**, 1079–81.
R36  Stewart J. *et al.* 1984. Does a water soluble contrast enema assist in the management of acute large bowel obstruction: a prospective study of 117 cases. *Br. J. Surg.* **71**, 799–801.
R37  Gilchrist A. *et al.* 1985. Acute large-bowel pseudo-obstruction. *Clin. Radiol.* **36**, 401–4.
R38  Millward S. *et al.* 1985. The barium enema appearances in solitary rectal ulcer syndrome. *Clin. Radiol.* **36**, 185–9.
R39  Fielding J. 1977. Irritable Bowel Syndrome: Clinical spectrum. *Clin. Gastroenterol.* **6**, 607–21.
R40  Rice R. *et al.* 1982. The diagnosis and significance of extra-luminal gas in the abdomen. *Radiol. Clin. North Am.* **20**, 819–37.
R41  Chapman R.W. *et al.* 1980. Primary sclerosing cholangitis: a review of its clinical features, cholangiography and hepatic histology. *Gut* **21**, 870–7.

# References

R42 Mueller P. & Simeone J. 1984. New concepts in biliary ultrasound. *Semin. Ultrasound.* **5**, 333–48.

R43 Bouchier I. 1983. Biochemistry of gallstone formation. *Clin. Gastroenterol.* **12**, 25–48.

R44 Eggert A. 1982. The pathologic implication of duodenal diverticula. *Surg. Gynaecol. Obstet.* **154**, 62–4.

R45 Kane R. & Katz S. 1982. The spectrum of sonographic findings in portal hypertension: a subject review and new observations. *Radiology* **142**, 453–8.

R46 Bolondi L. et al. 1982. Ultrasonography in the diagnosis of portal hypertension: diminished response of portal vessels to respiration. *Radiology* **142**, 167–72.

R47 Barter S. et al. 1985. Comparative studies of non-invasive investigation of Budd-Chiari syndrome. *Gut* **26**, A568.

R48 Powell-Jackson P. et al. 1985. Diagnosis of Budd-Chiari syndrome by liver US and colloid scintigraphy. *Gut* **26**, A568.

R49 Baert A. et al. 1983. Early diagnosis of Budd-Chiari syndrome by CT and US: report of 5 cases. *Gastroenterology* **84**, 587–95.

R50 Itai Y. et al. 1983. CT and sonography of cavernous haemangioma of the liver. *Am. J. Roentgenol* **141**, 315–20.

R51 Taboury J. et al. 1983. Cavernous haemangiomas of the liver studied by ultrasound. *Radiology* **149**, 781–5.

R52 Engel M. et al. 1983. Differentiation of focal intrahepatic lesions with Tc-red blood cell imaging. *Radiology* **146**, 777–82.

R53 Samuels B. et al. 1983. A comparison of radionuclide hepato-biliary imaging and real-time ultrasound for the detection of acute cholecystitis. *Radiology* **147**, 207–10.

R54 Drane W. et al. 1984. The need for routine delayed radionuclide hepatobiliary imaging in patients with severe intercurrent disease. *Radiology* **151**, 763–9.

R55 Gerhold J. et al. 1983. Diagnosis of biliary atresia with radionuclide hepatobiliary imaging. *Radiology* **146**, 499.

R56 Zeman R. et al. 1984. Strategy for the use of biliary scintigraphy in non-iatrogenic biliary trauma. *Radiology* **151**, 771–7.

R57 Durrell C. et al. 1984. Gallbladder sonography in clinical context. *Semin. Ultrasound.* **5**, 315–32.

R58 Ackery D. 1983. In: *Clinical Nuclear Medicine.* Ed. Maisey M.N., Britton K.E. & Gilday D.L. Chapman & Hall, London.

R59 Rhys Davies E. 1984. Radionuclide investigation. *Clin. Gastroenterol.* **13**, 205–33.

R60 Darlak J. et al. 1980. Calcifications in the liver. *Radiol. Clin. North Am.* **18**, 209.

R61 Federle M. & Burke V. 1984. Pancreatitis and its complications: Computed tomography and sonography. *Semin. Ultrasound.* **5**, 414–27.

R62 Gerzof S. et al. 1984. Percutaneous drainage of infected pancreatic pseudocysts. *Arch. Surg.* **119**, 888–93.

R63 Millward S. et al. 1983. Do plain films of the chest and abdomen have a role in the diagnosis of acute pancreatitis? *Clin. Radiol.* **34**, 133–7.

R64 Ring E. et al. 1973. Differential diagnosis of pancreatic calcification. *Am. J. Roentgenol.* **117**, 446–52.

R65 Nolan D. & Marks C. 1981. The barium infusion in small intestinal obstruction. *Clin. Radiol.* **32**, 657.

R66 Harned R. et al. 1982. Barium enema examination following biopsy of the rectum or colon. *Radiology* **145**, 11–16.

R67 Kreel L. 1978. Glucagon in Radiology. In: *Glucagon in Gastroenterology.* Ed. Picazo J. MTP Press Ltd, Lancaster.

R68 Watt I. & Middlemiss H. 1975. The radiology of gout. *Clin. Radiol.* **26**, 27–36.

R69 Edeiken J. 1982. Radiologic approach to arthritis. *Semin. Roentgenol.* **17**, 8–15.

R70 Forrester D., Brown J. & Nesson J. 1978. *The Radiology of Joint Disease.* 2nd Edition. W.B. Saunders, Philadelphia.

R71 Rabinowitz J. et al. 1974. Similar bone manifestations of scleroderma and rheumatoid arthritis. *Am. J. Roentgenol.* **121**, 35–44.

R72 Hamilton S. & Knickerbocker W. 1982. Peri-articular erosions in the hands and wrists in haemodialysis patients. *Clin. Radiol.* **33**, 19.

R73 Bywaters E. 1975. Jaccoud's syndrome. *Clin. Rheumatic Dis.* **1**, 125–48.

R74 Martel W. et al. 1979. Radiologic features of Reiter's disease. *Radiology* **132**, 1–10.

R75 Goldman A.B. 1982. Some miscellaneous joint diseases. *Semin. Roentgenol.* **17**, 60–80.

R76 Martel W. et al. 1980. Erosive osteoarthritis and psoriatic arthritis. *Am. J. Roentgenol.* **134**, 125–35.

R77 Kerr R. & Resnick D. 1985. Radiology of the seronegative spondyloarthropathies. *Clin. Rheumatic Dis.* **11**, 113–46.

R78 Resnick D. & Niwayama G. 1983. Entheses and Enthesopathy. *Radiology* **146**, 1–9.

R79 Petersdorf R.G. et al. (eds) 1983. *Harrison's Principles of Internal Medicine.* 10th Edition. McGraw-Hill, Maidenhead.

R80 Schumacher T. et al. 1978. HLA-B27 associated arthropathies. *Radiology* **126**, 289–97.

R81 Nance E.P. & Kaye J.J. 1982. The rheumatoid variants. *Semin. Roentgenol.* **17**, 16–24.

R82 Shearman D.J. & Finlayson N.D. 1982. *Diseases of the Gastrointestinal Tract and Liver.* Churchill Livingstone, Edinburgh.

R83 Calin A. 1985. Ankylosing spondylitis. *Clin. Rheumatic Dis.* **11**, 41–60.

R84 Jajic I. 1982. Gout in the spine and sacroiliac joints: Radiological manifestations. *Skeletal Radiol.* **8**, 209–12.

R85 Bonavita J.A. et al. 1980. Hydroxyapatite deposition disease. *Radiology* **134**, 621.

R86 Dalinka M.K. et al. 1982. Calcium deposition diseases. *Semin. Roentgenol.* **17**, 46.

R87 Martel W. et al. 1981. Further observations on the arthropathy of calcium pyrophosphate crystal deposition disease. *Radiology* **141**, 1–15.

R88 Greenfield G. 1980. *Radiology of Bone Diseases.* 3rd Edition. J.B. Lippincott, Philadelphia.

# References 199

**R89** Edeiken J. *et al.* 1967. Bone ischaemia. *Radiol. Clin. North Am.* **5**, 515–29.
**R90** Allen A.H. *et al.* 1978. The radiological changes in infections of the spine and their diagnostic value. *Clin. Radiol.* **29**, 31–40.
**R91** Chapman M. *et al.* 1979. Tuberculosis of bones and joints *Semin. Roentgenol.* **14**, 266–70.
**R92** Goldblatt M. & Cremin B. 1978. Osteo-articular tuberculosis: its presentation in coloured races. *Clin. Radiol.* **29**, 669–77.
**R93** Subbarao K. & Jacobbson H. 1979. Primary malignant neoplasms (of spine). *Semin. Roentgenol.* **14**, 44–57.
**R94** Dahlin D. 1978. *Bone tumours.* 3rd Edition. Charles C. Thomas, Springfield, Illinois.
**R95** Beabout J. *et al.* 1979. Benign tumours (of the spinal column). *Semin. Roentgenol.* **14**, 33–43.
**R96** Ennis J. *et al.* 1973. The radiology of the bone changes in Histiocytosis X. *Clin. Radiol.* **24**, 212–20.
**R97** Dahlin D. & McLeod R. 1972. Aneurysmal bone cyst and other non-neoplastic conditions. *Skeletal Radiol.* **8**, 243–50.
**R98** Gibson M. & Middlemiss J.H. 1971. Fibrous dysplasia of bone. *Br. J. Radiol.* **44**, 1–13.
**R99** Warrick C.K. 1973. Some aspects of polyostotic fibrous dysplasia. *Clin. Radiol.* **24**, 125–38.
**R100** Smith R. 1979. *Biochemical Disorders of the Skeleton.* Butterworths, London.
**R101** MacCarthy J. & Carey M. 1968. Bone changes in homocystinuria. *Clin. Radiol.* **19**, 128–34.
**R102** Cockshott P. & Middlemiss H. 1979. *Clinical Radiology in the Tropics.* Churchill Livingstone, Edinburgh.
**R103** Klatte E. *et al.* 1976. The radiographic spectrum in neuro-fibromatosis. *Semin. Roentgenol.* **11**, 17–33.
**R104** Leeds N. & Jacobson H. 1976. Spinal neurofibromatosis. *Am. J. Roentgenol.* **126**, 617–23.
**R105** Cope J. 1974. Carpal coalition. *Clin. Radiol.* **24**, 261–6.
**R106** Taybi H. 1983. *Radiology of Syndromes and Metabolic Disorders.* 2nd Edition. Year Book Medical Publishers, Chicago, Illinois.
**R107** James R. *et al.* 1972. The roentgenologic aspects of metastatic phaeochromocytoma. *Am. J. Roentgenol.* **115**, 783–93.
**R108** Steiner G. & Macdonald J. 1972. Metastases to bone from malignant melanoma. *Clin. Radiol.* **23**, 53–7.
**R109** Forbes G. *et al.* 1977. Radiographic manifestations of bone metastases from renal carcinoma. *Am. J. Roentgenol.* **129**, 61–6.
**R110** Beggs I. & Stoker D. 1982. Chondromyxoid fibroma of bone. *Clin. Radiol.* **33**, 671–9.
**R111** Bloem J. & Mulder J. 1985. Chondroblastoma: a clinical and radiological study of 104 cases. *Skeletal Radiol.* **14**, 1–9.
**R112** McLeod R. *et al.* 1976. The spectrum of osteoblastoma. *Am. J. Roentgenol.* **126**, 321–35.
**R113** Swee R. *et al.* 1979. Osteoid osteoma: Detection, diagnosis and localization. *Radiology* **130**, 117–23.
**R114** Shapiro F. 1982. Ollier's disease. *J. Bone Joint Surg.* **64A**, 95–103.

R115 Bonakdarpour A. *et al*. 1978. Primary and secondary aneurysmal bone cyst: a radiological study of 75 cases. *Radiology* **126**, 75–83.

R116 Jacobs P. 1972. The diagnosis of osteoclastoma (giant cell tumour): a radiological and pathological correlation. *Br. J. Radiol*. **1972**, 121–36.

R117 Capanna R. *et al*. 1985. Juxtaepiphyseal aneurysmal bone cyst. *Skeletal Radiol*. **13**, 21–5.

R118 Blaquiere R. *et al*. 1982. Sclerotic bone deposits in multiple myeloma. *Br. J. Radiol*. **55**, 591–3.

R119 Gompels B. *et al*. 1972. Correlation of radiological manifestations of multiple myeloma with immunoglobulin abnormalities and prognosis. *Radiology* **104**, 509–14.

R120 Ludwig H. *et al*. 1982. Radiography and bone scintigraphy in multiple myeloma — a comparative analysis. *Br. J. Radiol*. **55**, 173–81.

R121 Bataille R. *et al*. 1982. Bone scintigraphy in plasma-cell myeloma. *Radiology* **145**, 801–4.

R122 Levine E. *et al*. 1985. Juxtacortical osteosarcoma: a radiologic and histologic spectrum. *Skeletal Radiol*. **14**, 38–46.

R123 Hudson T. *et al*. 1983. Radiologic imaging of osteosarcoma: role in planning surgical treatment. *Skeletal Radiol*. **10**, 137–46.

R124 Pitt M. 1981. Rachitic and osteomalacic syndromes. *Radiol Clin. North Am*. **19**, 581–99.

R125 Kingston S. 1983. The role of Technetium and Gallium imaging in musculoskeletal disorders. *Clin. Rheumatic. Dis*. **9**, 347–85.

R126 Bassett L. *et al*. 1981. Radionuclide bone imaging. *Radiol. Clin. North Am*. **19**, 675–702.

R127 Heck L. 1984. Gamut: Extra-osseous localization of phosphate bone agents. *Semin. Nucl. Med*. **14**, 48–9.

R128 Caporn N. *et al*. 1983. Arthritis in Behcet's syndrome. *Br. J. Radiol*. **56**, 87–91.

R129 Guyer P. 1980. Radiology in Paget's disease. *Hospital Update* (Nov.) 1079–91.

R130 Frame B. & Marel G. 1981. Paget's disease: a review of current knowledge. *Radiology* **141**, 21–4.

R131 Dunn V. *et al*. 1981. Infants of diabetic mothers: radiographic manifestations. *Am. J. Roentgenol*. **37**, 123–8.

R132 Jacobson H. 1985. Dense bone — Too much bone: radiological considerations and differential diagnosis. Part 1. *Skeletal Radiol*. **13**, 1–20.

R133 Kattan K. Thickening of the heel pad associated with long-term Dilantin therapy. *Am. J. Radiol*. **124**, 52–6.

R134 Kho K. *et al*. 1970. Heel pad thickness in acromegaly. *Br. J. Radiol*. **43**, 119–25.

R135 Sherwood T. 1980. *Uroradiology*. Blackwell Scientific Publications, Oxford.

R136 Lalli A. 1982. Renal parenchymal calcifications. *Semin. Roentgenol*. **17**, 101–12.

R137 Davidson A. 1977. *Radiologic Diagnosis of Renal Parenchymal Disease*. W.B. Saunders, Philadelphia.

R138 Hare W. & Poynter J.D. 1974. The radiology of renal papillary necrosis as seen in analgesic nephropathy. *Clin. Radiol*. **25**, 423–43.

# References

R139 Hartman G. & Hodson C. 1969. The duplex kidney and related abnormalities. *Clin. Radiol.* **20**, 387–400.

R140 Braun B. *et al.* 1981. Ultrasonographic diagnosis of renal vein thrombosis. *Radiology* **138**, 157–8.

R141 Clark R. *et al.* 1979. Renal vein thrombosis: an underdiagnosed complication of multiple renal abnormalities. *Radiology* **132**, 43–50.

R142 Van Arsdalen K. 1984. Pathogenesis of renal calculi. *Urol. Radiol.* **6**, 65–73.

R143 Lang E. *et al.* 1984. Angio-CT and dynamic CT in staging of renal cell carcinoma. *Radiology* **151**, 149–55.

R144 Madewell J. 1979. Radiologic-pathologic correlations in cystic disease of the kidney. *Radiol. Clin. North Am.*, **17**, 261–79.

R145 Mena F. *et al.* 1973. Neurofibromatosis and renovascular hypertension in children. *Am. J. Roentgenol.* **118**, 39–45.

R146 Kirks D. *et al.* 1981. Diagnostic imaging of pediatric abdominal masses: an overview. *Radiol. Clin. North Am.* **19**, 527–45.

R147 Lowe P. & Roylance J. 1976. Transitional cell carcinoma of the kidney. *Clin. Radiol.* **27**, 503–12.

R148 Elkin M. 1975. Renal cystic disease: an overview. *Semin. Roentgenol.* **10**, 99–102.

R149 Takebayashi S. 1985. Acquired cystic disease on dialysis. *Urol. Radiol.* **7**, 69–74.

R150 Bosniak M. & Ambos M. 1975. Polycystic kidney disease. *Semin. Roentgenol.* **10**, 133–43.

R151 Whitehouse G.H. 1975. Some urographic aspects of the horseshoe kidney anomaly — a review of 59 cases. *Clin. Radiol.* **26**, 107–14.

R152 Lang E. 1975. Roentgenologic assessment of medullary cysts. *Semin. Roentgenol.* **10**, 145–54.

R153 Editorial 1985. Xanthogranulomatous pyelonephritis. *Lancet* ii 649–50.

R154 Cremin B. 1979. Observations on vesico-ureteric reflux and intrarenal reflux: a review and survey of material. *Clin. Radiol.* **30**, 607–21.

R155 Dixon A. *et al.* 1984. Computed tomographic observations in periaortitis: a hypothesis. *Clin. Radiol.* **35**, 39–42.

R156 Minford J. & Davies P. 1984. The urographic appearances in acute and chronic retroperitoneal fibrosis. *Clin. Radiol.* **35**, 51–7.

R157 Fagan C. *et al.* 1982 Retroperitoneal fibrosis. *Semin. Ultrasound* **3**, 123–38.

R158 Desai S., Eliot C. & Lawton G. 1985. Bladder shape and racial origin. *Clin. Radiol.* **36**, 377–8.

R159 Ambros M. *et al.* 1977. The pear-shaped bladder. *Radiology* **122**, 85–8.

R160 Friedenberg R. 1983. Abnormalities affecting structure and function of the bladder and urethra. *Semin. Roentgenol.* **18**, 307–21.

R161 Adam E. *et al.* 1985. Racial variations in normal ureteric course. *Clin. Radiol.* **36**, 373–5.

R162 Graham D. & Sanders R. 1982. Amniotic fluid. *Semin. Roentgenol.* **17**, 210–8.

R163 Moore P. *et al.* 1984. Sonographic diagnosis of hydramnios and oligohydramnios. *Semin. Ultrasound* **5**, 157–69.

**R164** Pasto M. & Kurtz A. 1984. The prenatal examination of the fetal cranium, spine and CNS. *Semin. Ultrasound* **5**, 170–93.
**R165** Makuno D. *et al.* 1984. Sonography of the fetal gastrointestinal system. *Semin. Ultrasound* **5**, 194–209.
**R166** Spirt B. *et al.* 1982. The placenta: sonographic-pathological correlations. *Semin. Roentgenol.* **17**, 219–30.
**R167** Jeanty P. & Romero R. 1984. Estimation of the gestational age. *Semin. Ultrasound* **5**, 121–9.
**R168** Romero R. and Jeanty P. 1984. The detection of fetal growth disorders. *Semin. Ultrasound* **5**, 130–43.
**R169** Whitehouse G.H. 1981. *Gynaecological Radiology*. Blackwell Scientific Publications, Oxford.
**R170** Lewis E. *et al.* 1982. Radiologic contributions to the diagnosis and management of gynecologic neoplasms. *Semin. Roentgenol.* **17**, 251–68.
**R171** Deutsch A. & Gosink B. 1982. Non-neoplastic gynecologic disorders. *Semin. Roentgenol.* **17**, 269–83.
**R172** Heitzman E., Markarian B. & Solomon J. 1973. Chronic obstructive pulmonary disease. *Radiol. Clin. North Am.* **11**, 49–75.
**R173** Simon G. 1970. Radiology and chronic airways obstruction. In: *Modern Trends in Diagnostic Radiology — 4*. Ed. McLaren J. Butterworths, London.
**R174** Thurlbeck W. & Simon G. 1978. Radiographic appearance of the chest in emphysema. *Am. J. Roentgenol.* **130**, 429–40.
**R175** Gishen P. *et al.* 1982. Alpha-1-antitrypsin deficiency: the radiological features of pulmonary emphysema in subjects of Pi type Z and Pi type SZ. *Clin. Radiol.* **33**, 371–7.
**R176** Hodson C. & France N. 1962. Pulmonary changes in cystic fibrosis of the pancreas. A radio-pathological study. *Clin. Radiol.* **13**, 54.
**R177** Friedman P. *et al.* 1981. Pulmonary cystic fibrosis in the adult: early and late radiologic findings with pathologic correlation. *Am. J. Roentgenol.* **136**, 131–1144.
**R178** Fraser R.G. & Pare J.A.P. 1979. *Diagnosis of Diseases of the Chest*. 2nd Edition. Saunders, Philadelphia.
**R179** James D.G. & Carstairs L.S. 1982. Pulmonary sarcoidosis. *Hospital Update* 1982, 1022–30.
**R180** Freundlich I. *et al.* 1970. Sarcoidosis. Typical and atypical thoracic manifestations and complications. *Clin. Radiol.* **21**, 376–83.
**R181** Kirks D., McCormick V. & Greenspan R. 1973. Pulmonary sarcoidosis: Roentgenologic analysis of 150 patients. *Am. J. Roentgenol.* **117**, 777–86.
**R182** Morrison D. & Goldman A. 1979. Radiographic patterns of drug-induced lung disease. *Radiology* **131**, 299.
**R183** Sostman H. *et al.* 1981. Diagnosis of chemotherapy lung. *Am. J. Roentgenol.* **136**, 33–40.
**R184** Hargreave F. *et al.* 1972. The radiological appearances of allergic alveolitis due to bird sensitivity. *Clin. Radiol.* **23**, 1–10.
**R185** Pierce J. & Kerr I. 1978. Immunologic diseases and the lung. *Radiol. Clin. North Am.* **16**, 389–406.
**R186** Greene R. 1981. The pulmonary aspergilloses: three distinct entities or a spectrum of disease. *Radiology* **140**, 527–30.

**R187** Phelan M. & Kerr I. 1984. Allergic broncho-pulmonary aspergillosis: the radiological appearances during long-term follow-up. *Clin. Radiol.* **35**, 385–92.
**R188** Schatz M. 1979. Immunologic lung disease. *New Eng. J. Med.* **300**, 1310–20.
**R189** Weber A. *et al.* 1965. Roentgenologic patterns in longstanding beryllium disease. *Am. J. Roentgenol.* **93**, 879–90.
**R190** Soutar C. *et al.* 1974. The radiology of asbestos-induced disease of the lungs. *Br. J. Dis. Chest* **68**, 235–52.
**R191** Galloway R. 1984. Problems in asbestos related disease. *Rachiol. Now* **2**, 8.
**R192** Greening R. & Heslep J. 1967. The roentgenology of silicosis. *Semin. Roentgenol.* **2**, 265–75.
**R193** Dee P. *et al.* 1979. Pneumocystis carinii infection of the lung: radiological and pathological correlation. *Am. J. Roentgenol.* **132**, 741–6.
**R194** Greene R. 1980. Opportunistic pneumonias. *Semin. Roentgenol.* **15**, 50–72.
**R195** Heitzman E. 1977. Bronchogenic carcinoma: Radiologic-pathologic correlations. *Semin. Roentgenol.* **12**, 165–74.
**R196** Greene R. *et al.* 1977. Other malignant tumours of the lung. *Semin. Roentgenol.* **12**, 225.
**R197** Hill C.A. 1984. Bronchioalveolar carcinoma: a review. *Radiology* **150**, 15–20.
**R198** Dunnick W. *et al.* 1976. Rapid onset of pulmonary infiltration due to histiocytic lymphoma. *Radiology* **118**, 281–5.
**R199** Blank N. & Castellino R. 1980. The intrathoracic manifestions of the malignant lymphomas and the leukaemias. *Semin. Roentgenol.* **15**, 227–45.
**R200** Trapnell D. 1963. The peripheral lymphatics of the lungs. *Br. J. Radiol.* **63**, 660–72.
**R201** Felson B. 1979. A new look at pattern recognition of diffuse pulmonary disease. *Am. J. Roentgenol.* **133**, 183–9.
**R202** Sullivan D. *et al.* 1983. Lung scan interpretation: effect of different observers and different criteria. *Radiology* **149**, 803–7.
**R203** Thomason C. & Rao B.R. 1983. Lung imaging — unilateral absence or near absence of pulmonary perfusion on lung scanning. *Semin. Nucl. Med.* **13**, 388.
**R204** Neumann R. *et al.* 1980. Current status of ventilation-perfusion imaging. *Semin. Nucl. Med.* **10**, 198–217.
**R205** Hublitz U. & Shapiro J. 1974. The radiology of pulmonary oedema. *Crit. Rev. Clin. Radiol.* **5**, 389–422.
**R206** Calenoff L. *et al.* 1978. Unilateral pulmonary edema. *Radiology* **126**, 19–24.
**R207** Singleton E. 1981. Radiologic consideration of intensive care in the premature infant. *Radiology* **140**, 291–300.
**R208** Choplin R. & Siegel M. 1980. Pulmonary sequestration: six unusual presentations. *Am. J. Roentgenol.* **134**, 695–700.
**R209** Maile C. *et al.* 1982. Calcification in pulmonary metastases. *Br. J. Radiol.* **55**, 108–13.
**R210** Siegelman S. *et al.* 1984. Computed tomography of the solitary pulmonary nodule. *Semin. Roentgenol.* **19**, 165–72.
**R211** Schulman A. *et al.* 1982. Air in unusual places: some causes and ramifications of pneumomediastinum. *Clin. Radiol.* **33**, 301–6.

R212 Greene R. et al. 1977. Pneumothorax. *Semin. Roentgenol.* **12**, 313–25.
R213 McLoud T. & Meyer J. 1982. Mediastinal metastases. *Radiol. Clin. North Am.* **20**, 453–68.
R214 Day D. & Gedaudas E. 1984. The Thymus. *Radiol. Clin. North Am.* **22**, 519–38.
R215 Goodman L. & Putman C. 1981. The S.I.C.U. chest radiograph after massive blunt trauma. *Radiol. Clin. North Am.* **19**, 111–23.
R216 Bissett G. & Meyer M. 1983. Obstructive left heart lesions. *Semin. Roentgenol.* **20**, 244–53.
R217 Van Praagh R. 1985. The importance of segmental situs in the diagnosis of congenital heart disease. *Semin. Roentgenol.* **20**, 254–71.
R218 Shinebourne E. *et al.* 1976. Sequential chamber localization — logical approach to diagnosis in congenital heart disease. *Br. Heart J.* **38**, 237–340.
R219 Green C. *et al.* 1985. Atrial septal defect. *Semin. Roentgenol.* **20**, 214–25.
R220 Soto B. *et al.* 1985. Ventricular septal defect. *Semin. Roentgenol.* **20**, 200–13.
R221 Jefferson K. & Rees S. 1980. *Clinical Cardiac Radiology*. 2nd Edition, Butterworths, London.
R222 Smith C. *et al.* 1979. Tricuspid and pulmonary valves: Combined valvular disease. *Semin. Roentgenol.* **14**, 144–52.
R223 Swischuk L. 1985. Patent ductus arteriosus. *Semin. Roentgenol.* **20**, 236–43.
R224 Goodwin J. 1979. A current appraisal of the cardiomyopathies. *Hospital Update* 665.
R225 Editorial 1979. The floppy mitral valve. *Lancet* **i**, 138.
R226 Chan F. *et al.* 1983. Skeletal abnormalities in mitral-valve prolapse. *Clin. Radiol.* **34**, 207.
R227 Lyons K. *et al.* 1980. Pyrophosphate myocardial imaging. *Semin. Nucl. Med.* **10**, 168–77.
R228 Pohost G. *et al.* 1980. Thallium redistribution: mechanisms and clinical utility. *Semin. Nucl. Med.* **10**, 70–93.
R229 Carsky E. *et al.* 1980. The epicardial fat pad sign. *Radiology* **137**, 303–8.
R230 Newell J., Higgins C. & Kelley M. 1980. Radiographic–echocardiographic approach to acquired heart disease: diagnosis and assessment of severity. *Radiol. Clin. North Am.* **18**, 387–409.
R231 Godwin J. & Korobkin M. 1983. Acute disease of the aorta: Diagnosis by CT and US. *Radiol. Clin. North Am.* **21**, 551–74.
R232 Dee P. *et al.* 1985. The CT and Ultrasound diganosis of aortic dissection. *Semin. Ultrasound* **6**, 146–55.
R233 Ang J. 1983. Gamut: Renal microaneurysms (including necrotizing angiitis). *Semin. Roentgenol.* **18**, 169–70.
R234 Streiter M. & Bosniak M. 1983. The radiology of drug addiction: urinary tract complications. *Semin. Roentgenol.* **18**, 221–6.
R235 Woodring J. *et al.* 1984. Mediastinal haemorrhage: an evaluation of radiographic manifestations. *Radiology* **151**, 15.
R236 Heiberg E. & Wolverson M. 1985. CT of traumatic injuries of the aorta. *Semin. Ultrasound* **6**, 172–80.

# References

R237 Fisher R. et al. 1981. Laceration of the thoracic aorta and brachiocephalic arteries by blunt trauma. *Radiol. Clin. North Am.* **19**, 91–110.

R238 Boyez M. 1982. Case of the winter season: Mycotic aneurysms complicating bacterial endocarditis. *Semin. Roentgenol.* **17**, 5–7.

R239 Kaufman S. et al. 1978. Protean manifestation of mycotic aneurysms. *Am. J. Roentgenol.* **131**, 1019–25.

R240 De Boulay G. (Ed.) 1984. *A textbook of Radiological Diagnosis.* Vol 1. 5th Edition. H.K. Lewis, London.

R241 Lloyd G. 1975. *Radiology of the Orbit.* W.B. Saunders, Philadelphia.

R242 Bydder G. et al. 1983. NMR imaging of the posterior fossa: 50 cases. *Clin. Radiol.* **34**, 173–88.

R243 Bradley W. et al. 1984. Comparison of CT and MR in 400 patients with suspected disease of the brain and cervical spinal cord. *Radiology* **152**, 195–202.

R244 Brant-Zawadzki M. et al. 1983 NMR demonstration of cerebral abnormalities: comparison with CT. *Am. J. Roentgenol.* **140**, 847–854.

R245 Han J. et al. 1984. Head trauma evaluated by MR and CT: a comparison. *Radiology* **150**, 71–7.

R246 Bydder G. 1984. MRI of the brain. *Radiol. Clin. North Am.* **22**, 779.

R247 Rosenbaum A. & Rosenbloom S. 1984 Meningiomas revisited. *Semin. Roentgenol.* **19**, 8–26.

R248 Leeds N. et al. 1984. Gliomas of the brain. *Semin. Roentgenol.* **19**, 27–43.

R249 Coulam C. et al. 1976. Von Hippel Landau syndrome. *Semin. Roentgenol.* **11**, 61–6.

R250 Coulam C. et al. 1976. Sturge-Weber syndrome. *Semin. Roentgenol.* **11**, 55–60.

R251 Kerfkins R. et al. 1984. Magnetic resonance imaging of the internal auditory canal. *Radiology* **151**, 105–8.

R252 Pinto R. & Kricheff I. 1984. Neuroradiology of intracranial neuromas. *Semin. Roentgenol.* **19**, 44–52.

R253 Moseley I. 1981. Aneurysms of the cerebral arteries. *Br. J.H.M.* **26**, 612–8.

R254 Davis K. et al. 1982. A neuroradiological approach to the patient with a clinical diagnosis of subarachnoid haemorrhage. *Radiol. Clin. North Am.* **20**, 87–94.

R255 Hankins C.A. et al. 1985. Prolactinomas: Clinical presentation, radiologic assessment, and therapeutic options. *Invest. Radiol.* **20**, 345–54.

R256 Hattery R.R. et al. 1981. Computed tomography of the adrenal gland. *Semin. Roentgenol.* **16**, 290.

R257 Johnson C. et al. 1985. CT of the adrenal cortex. *Semin. Ultrasound* **6**, 241–60.

R258 Sutton D. 1975. The radiological diagnosis of adrenal tumours. *Br. J. Radiol.* **48**, 237–58.

R259 Johnson C. et al. 1985. CT of the adrenal medulla. *Semin. Ultrasound* **6**, 219–40.

R260 Dodd G. 1985. The radiological features of Multiple Endocrine Neoplasia Types IIA and IIB. *Semin. Roentgenol.* **20**, 64–90.

R261 James E.M. & Charboneau J. 1985. High-frequency (10 MHz) thyroid ultrasonography. *Semin. Ultrasound* **6**, 294–309.

R262 Stark D. *et al.* 1985. Non-invasive parathyroid imaging. *Semin. Ultrasound* **6**, 310–20.
R263 Doppmann J. 1985. Overview: Multiple endocrine syndromes — a nightmare for the endocrinologic radiologist. *Semin. Roentgenol.* **20**, 7–16.
R264 Dodds W. *et al.* 1985. MEN I syndrome and islet cell lesions of the pancreas. *Semin. Roentgenol.* **20**, 17–63.
R265 Segel M. *et al.* 1984. Diabetes mellitus: the predominant cause of bilateral renal enlargement. *Radiology* **153**, 341–2.
R266 Raval B. & Lamki N. 1985. Computed tomography of the traumatized abdomen. *Semin. Ultrasound* **6**, 109–28.
R267 Gelfand M. 1984. Scintigraphy in upper abdominal trauma. *Semin. Roentgenol.* **19**, 296–307.
R268 Dodd G. & Jing B-S. 1977. In: Radiology of the nose, paranasal sinuses and nasopharynx. Section 2, *Golden's Diagnostic Radiology*. William & Wilkins, Baltimore.
R269 Som P. *et al.* 1982. The angiomatous polyp and the angiofibroma: 2 different lesions. *Radiology* **144**, 329–34.
R270 Stern W. & Subbarao K. 1983. Pulmonary complications of drug addiction. *Semin. Roentgenol.* **18**, 183–97.
R271 Firooznia H. *et al.* 1983. Radiology of musculoskeletal complications of drug addiction. *Semin. Roentgenol.* **18**, 198–206.
R272 Jaffe R. 1983. Cardiac and vascular involvement in drug abuse. *Semin. Roentgenol.* **18**, 207–12.
R273 Balthazar E. & Lefleur R. 1983. Abdominal complications of drug addiction. *Semin. Roentgenol.* **18**, 198–206.
R274 Streiter M. & Bosniak M. 1983. The radiology of drug addiction: urinary tract complications. *Semin. Roentgenol.* **18**, 221–6.
R275 Leeds N. *et al.* 1983. The radiology of drug addiction affecting the brain. *Semin. Roentgenol.* **18**, 227–33.
R276 Epstein B. 1976. *The Spine: A Radiological Text and Atlas*. 4th Edition. Lea and Febiger, Philadelphia.
R277 Wolfe J.N. 1972. *Xeroradiography of the Breast*. Charles C. Thomas, Springfield, Illinois.